GITA 3

A CONTEMPORARY GUIDE TO
THE TIMELESS TEACHINGS OF
THE BHAGAVAD-GITA

B.B. Keshava Swami

The International Society for Krishna Consciousness
Founder Acarya: His Divine Grace A.C. Bhaktivedanta Swami Prabhupada

www.keshavaswami.com
www.schoolofbhakti.com
www.thinkgita.org

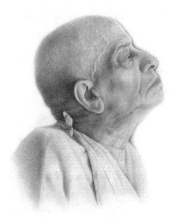

The Inspiration

A.C. Bhaktivedanta Swami Prabhupada was a saint like no other. In 1966, at the age of 69, homeless, penniless and alone, he arrived in the Lower East Side of New York, searching for 'better opportunities' to share the message of the Gita. This was Skid Row; the lowest of the low. Here he lived, worshiped, studied and taught. Every evening, his decrepit residence, the rat-ridden 94 Bowery, would fill up with buzzing acidheads, bearded bohemians, ruined alcoholics and disillusioned dropouts. Sex, music, LSD, and consciousness expansion; that's what made them tick. The Swami would nonchalantly step into the makeshift 'temple' and take his seat at the front, face-to-face with these confused souls who were looking for real love, real happiness and real spiritual experience.

The Swami was unfazed; his expression exuding bottomless depth and boundless compassion. In short, straight-forward philosophical discourses, he delivered eternal truths with resounding impact. When he sang in simple tunes with a bongo drum, their heads would spin, and their hearts would be conquered. His tremendous devotion empowered his urgent message to penetrate the depths of their consciousness. He effortlessly smashed layers of illusion, unrelentingly exposing the fallacy of all materialistic ideology.

From these humble beginnings, Prabhupada went on to establish the International Society for Krishna Consciousness (ISKCON), and in a few short years made 'Hare Krishna' a household name. He circled the globe twelve times, opened over a hundred temples, launched a variety of spiritual welfare projects, authored volumes of books, and made genuine spirituality inspiring, practical and accessible for people from all walks of life. No amount of social commentary, historical analysis or anthropological conjecture can account for his incredible achievements. Prabhupada's story is tangible proof of a spiritual miracle that defied all odds. His life and teachings remain the strength, inspiration and guiding light.

Gita3 is based on Srila Prabhupada's Bhagavad-gita As It Is, the world's most popular and widely read edition of the ancient classic. It has been translated in over sixty languages and is available in nearly every major city in the world.

Gratitude

My spiritual master, Kadamba Kanana Swami, who departed from the world in 2023, was the proof-reader of my life. He revealed a vision that extended way beyond my own limited perception, infusing me with the belief and empowerment to progress forward. Because he told me to write, I'm trying my best.

There are some individuals who have more faith in you than yourself. For me, the late Srutidharma Das was one of those people; an endless fountain of encouragement and empowerment. He was a living theology – the Bhagavad-gita in action.

Several kind-hearted individuals offered invaluable feedback, input and advice – Pranada Devi Dasi, Chris, Lila Kamala and Jenny. Thanks for your time and energy. Credit for the front cover design goes to Urvi. Finally, my gratitude to Yogi – a technical whizz kid who effortlessly transforms a manuscript into a printed book.

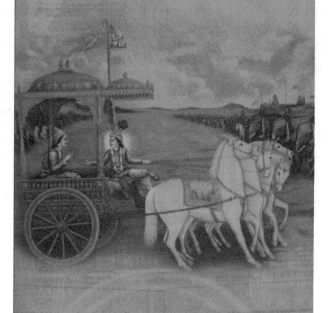

BHAGAVAD GĪTĀ AS IT IS

HIS DIVINE GRACE
A. C. BHAKTIVEDANTA SWAMI PRABHUPĀDA
Founder-*Ācārya* of the International Society for Krishna Consciousness

Introduction

After graduating from University College London in 2002, my life path was veering toward the default trajectory. Spiritual hunger, however, was drawing me into dangerous territory. My calling was different and I didn't want to live with regrets, but finding the courage to follow my heart wasn't easy. After two failed attempts, I somehow made a leap of faith and re-routed to the road less travelled. Third time lucky! I became a 21-year old monk, slept on the floor, rose before the sun, lived out of a locker, and made scriptural study, selfless service, and spiritual absorption my chosen career. No regrets. Over two decades later I continue to do the same, inspired and enthused, knowing that there is so much more to discover.

Third time lucky rings true indeed. Whether the chanting of *mantras*, circumambulations of holy objects, or the sequence in spiritual ceremonies, the magic number is definitely three. Aside from the esoteric and numerological explanations of the figure three, there is a very practical benefit. In today's age of mass distraction we need multiple attempts to bring our full attention to anything. Repeated efforts bring clarity, depth and conviction to any activity. In Gita3, we'll take you on a scenic journey through the spiritual landscape of the Bhagavad-gita... three times!

If we had to choose a single book to represent the spiritual wisdom of India, the Bhagavad-gita would surely top the list. In 700 power-packed verses it summarises the profound conclusions of the Vedas, the ancient scriptures written over 5000 years ago in the Sanskrit language. It's a theological and philosophical classic, and its scope is expansive. It covers everything from religion to relationships, science to sociology, leadership to lifestyle management: the keys to all aspects of life, the universe and everything. In every generation, over thousands of years, it has provided unceasing inspiration to thinkers, leaders, and seekers alike.

Since this classic was spoken by Krishna, the Supreme Person, it's no surprise that the timeless contents are so special. The Bhagavad-gita's insights are clear, concise, logical, and scientific – not just appealing to a particular faith, belief, or culture. Those who sincerely study and apply the wisdom will witness how its teachings transform one's entire being. That is why the Bhagavad-gita remains one of the most popular books in the world today - a perennial bestseller.

In Part One, entitled *'Think Different,'* we explore the Gita's paradigm-shifting principles, confronting and challenging the default worldviews instilled within us. We'll conduct a series of thought experiments to demonstrate the life-changing impact of these spiritual insights.

In Part Two, entitled *'How To,'* we'll share the Gita's tools and techniques, aimed at transforming us into the best version of ourselves. For each chapter there'll be life hacks and practical, step-by-step guidance on how to apply the principles and activate the transformation.

In Part Three, entitled *'Why Not,'* we'll witness how the justifications we offer to delay or deny our spiritual progress are nothing more than excuses. The sheer practicality of the Gita shines through, and we deep-dive into select verses which dissipate any lingering doubts.

Read on, pause for thought, let the simple but powerful philosophy enter your heart, and see how you begin to look at life differently. Read it from front to back or dive into a section which catches your interest. Cross reference the insights with the original Bhagavad-gita, discuss the passages with your friends, and experiment with the exercises. Allow us to share with you the principles, process, and practicality of the Bhagavad-gita. This is *wisdom that breathes.*

S.B. Keshava Swami

The Battlefield of Life

In the epic masterpiece, Mahabharata, the longest poem in the world, the history of ancient India is documented. The story, full of twists and turns, romance and tragedy, philosophy and poetry, reaches its climax at the onset of a devastating war between a family in feud.

Over 5000 years ago, innumerable troops had converged on Kurukshetra (90 miles north of present-day Delhi) for what was billed as the greatest battle ever. Through a series of intrigues and conspiracies, the evil-minded Kauravas had usurped the throne of the Pandavas. Though born in the same clan, the Kauravas (sons of Dhritarastra) and the Pandavas (sons of Pandu) were at polar opposites. The former were plagued by greed, selfishness and pride, whereas the saintly Pandavas were individuals of the highest moral stature, dedicated to virtue, devotion and righteousness. Though grossly exploited and mistreated, the Pandavas repeatedly sought amicable means to redress the injustice, but the stubborn and greedy Kauravas were unwilling to budge an inch. Military battle and a trial of arms was inevitable.

Arjuna, the talented and dynamic Pandava archer who carried a heavyweight burden of expectation, readied himself for a face-off. As tumultuous battle cries pervaded the air, the distinguished warrior suddenly experienced a moment of doubt. He requested Krishna, the Supreme Person who had assumed the position of a humble driver, to steer his chariot to the middle of the battlefield. There, Arjuna registered the reality before him – the inevitable suffering and death that would consume his family, friends, fellow countrymen and soldiers who had assembled on that battlefield.

This triggered an existential confusion! In desperation, Arjuna began asking questions he had never raised before. These were the 'big' questions, inquiries pertaining to the happiness we all so much seek. These are the questions which linger deep within us all, but remain unaddressed in most people's lifetime. A penetrating conversation with Krishna ensued, gems of invaluable wisdom surfaced, and the

Bhagavad-gita ('the song of God') was born.

The Gita was spoken to comfort, coach and convince Arjuna in his moment of weakness. Krishna's purpose, however, was much broader. On our own 'battlefield of life' we'll all encounter moments of confusion which prompt us to venture beyond the routine treadmill of life. The Bhagavad-gita presents timeless answers to those perennial questions, offering an opportunity to upgrade our life on every conceivable level. Ancient wisdom, eternally relevant.

References

For each chapter we have referenced specific verses from the Bhagavad-gita which will offer greater insight and inspiration. We encourage our readers to take full advantage of Gita3 by simultaneously referring to the *Bhagavad-gita As It Is*.

Part One: *Think Different*

*The Bhagavad-gita challenges the principles
which underpin our life.*

	World teaches	Gita teaches
1	Leave the Problems	Learn from Problems
2	Act First, Ask Later	Ask First, Act Later
3	Spiritualists don't Own	Spiritualists aren't Owned
4	Know through Study	Know through Sincerity
5	Be the Best	Try your Best
6	Train your Body	Train your Mind
7	See to Believe	Hear to See
8	Live Before you Die	Die Before you Die
9	Ask God for your Wants	Give God what He Wants
10	Can't See God Anywhere	Can See God Everywhere
11	Believe in Yourself	Believe in Krishna
12	Make a 'To-Do' list	Make a 'To-Be' list
13	God is Far, Seated in Heaven	God is Near, Seated Within
14	The Wealthy Have the Most	The Wealthy Need the Least
15	Pursue your Dreams	Discover the Reality
16	I, Me, and Mine	We, Us, and Ours
17	Faith Opposes Knowledge	Faith Builds Knowledge
18	Try to be Happy	Try to Serve

If someone tells a lie loud enough and long enough, others begin to accept it as truth. When enough people are convinced by that 'truth' it becomes a culture. If that culture is somehow transmitted to the next generation, it becomes a tradition. Such traditions, and the worldviews and behaviours they espouse, become etched into society, followed by millions, usually without question. Our weapons of mass instruction - educational systems, media powerhouses and community structures - reinforce these traditions, causing untruth to perpetuate over decades and centuries. Blind leading the blind, all completely oblivious to the illusion.

Amidst the mass of people are some unique individuals who begin to challenge what everyone else passively accepts. It takes courage to question, intelligence to search, and determination to change. Beware... going against the grain is risky business! It's much easier to go with the flow and tread the path of least resistance. The world has its preconceived notions - what's acceptable and what's not - and most people seamlessly fit right in. Yet some just can't. The excitement, intrigue and hunger to find out what lies beyond the 'safe' path in life drives them to embark on the road less travelled.

Over the centuries, philosophers, spiritualists, scientists and thinkers have discussed and debated with a view to understanding the world in a more profound way. The sages of the East were no different. In the ancient body of literatures known as the Vedas, they documented a spiritual understanding of the self, the universe and the deeper purpose in the journey of life. The essential truths they disclosed inspire one to break free from stereotypes and upgrade their existence. Endowed with such insights, one can flourish on all levels - physically, emotionally, socially, and most importantly, spiritually.

Read on, and discover how Krishna coaches Arjuna to approach the world in a way quite different to what we've been taught growing up. You can cheat some people all of the time, and all people some of the time. You can't, however, cheat all the people, all the time. The Bhagavad-gita launches a head-on challenge. Krishna invites us to think differently. We must resist the temptation to be 'normal,' because those who are now considered 'normal' accept the principles and practices of an insane world. *Are you ready to be different?*

LEAVE THE ① LEARN FROM
problems

The Bhagavad-gita opens with Arjuna, an esteemed and valiant fighter, undergoing an existential crisis. He requests Krishna, who has taken the humble position of being his driver, to draw his chariot to the middle of the battlefield. Before plunging into full-scale warfare, Arjuna wants to witness the formidable fighters who have assembled to engage in this historic trial of arms. Seeing his friends, family members and teachers, he becomes overwhelmed with emotion, contemplating the suffering and death that will inevitably transpire. Arjuna's body begins to tremble, his bow slips from his hand, his skin starts to burn, and, sweating in anxiety, his mind reels with conflicting thoughts. Completely displaced, he helplessly approaches Krishna and concedes: *"I can't bear this predicament - I need to leave the battlefield. I must change my situation."*

When faced with problems, our instinctive reaction is one of escape. It seems natural and logical to remove ourselves from the situation, create distance, seek relief, and mitigate the immediate discomfort. The default response is to make external adjustments to solve our problems. When relationships get rocky, it's easier to turn your back. When obstacles unexpectedly appear, we change our path or give up entirely. When situations demand sacrifice, we bow out and revert to the comfortable alternative. *Could it be, however, that every difficulty we encounter is meant to evolve, edify and elevate our consciousness? Could unwanted impediments be part of a master plan to usher us into a higher awareness of life? Perhaps challenges appear for our growth?*

In troublesome times, we shouldn't impulsively clutch for an external fix, but rather focus on nurturing internal growth. In difficulty, we often look up at God as victims and question, *"Why is this happening to me?"* Instead, we could look up as seekers and ask, *"How can I learn and grow from this?"* Everyone will *go* through problems, but the wise soul learns to *grow* through problems. If we instinctively eject ourselves from the difficult situations we encounter, failing to learn or evolve from them, the same situations will likely reappear again and again.

In the dialogue that ensues, Krishna encourages Arjuna to embrace his daunting task as a warrior. On the surface, Arjuna's arguments for opting out of battle seem credible, indeed even spiritual. Krishna, however, exposes Arjuna's weakness and discourages his proposed exit from the battlefield. Every event and experience appears for a reason. It's that reason, that lesson, that teaching, that we must decipher. Krishna assures Arjuna that this situation will provide him a unique opportunity to develop his spiritual consciousness. It's this spiritual consciousness that will provide immunity from the inescapable chaos of material life, and simultaneously connect one to the Supreme Person and eternal reality.

We each have our life path, and every journey is peppered with challenges. Though we may sometimes opt to adjust the externals and alter the practical dynamics, we should know that such changes are not solutions in and of themselves. Everything we encounter is meant to rewire our consciousness and renovate our inner world.

"I am now unable to stand here any longer. I am forgetting myself, and my mind is reeling. I see only causes of misfortune, O Krishna, killer of the Kesi demon."

(Bhagavad-gita 1.30)

References

1.30 – Arjuna's lack of spiritual vision brings fear and dejection.

2.9 – Arjuna puts down his bow and decides to retire from the battle.

Hidden Stories

Back Tracking

Think of a time when you went through a painful challenge or difficulty. Reflect on how your life has evolved since that time, and identify three positive things that came from it.

1.

2.

3.

Forward Facing

Think of an uncomfortable situation or problem you are currently facing. Can you reflect why you may be experiencing this and what lessons you could learn from it? If you learnt these lessons, how would your life improve?

Deja vu

Think of a recurring situation that you find yourself facing again and again - maybe a relationship struggle, a financial issue, a physical ailment or emotional challenge. Can you identify a lesson that you failed to learn which may be causing this to reappear?

Group Discussion: *How can we decipher the lesson we need to learn from any given situation?*

In the emotional chaos of life, it's often difficult for us to step away and appreciate how the situation at hand can aid us to upgrade our existence. With Krishna's encouragement, Arjuna embraced his situation and went on to flourish in all aspects of life. In hindsight, it's scary to think what may have happened if Arjuna had retired from the battlefield!

Learning the art of being an observer of life, and not just an invested participant, can transform everything.

ASK first ACT ②later ASK
ACT ACT

The urge to find pleasure drives everything we do. Capitalising on this universal urge, society has trained us to seek satisfaction through romance, sports, the arts, education, our professions and much more. Yet we're often left with feelings of dissatisfaction and emptiness. The Dalai Lama, when asked what surprised him most about humanity, answered *"Man! Because he sacrifices his health in order to make money. Then he sacrifices money to recuperate his health. And then he is so anxious about the future that he does not enjoy the present; the result being that he does not live in the present or the future; he lives as if he is never going to die, and then dies having never really lived."* Are we confused?

Before deciding where to invest time, resource and effort, a wise person clarifies their *purpose*. It seems logical to start with the question *"Why?"* Unfortunately, since we live in a world which is endlessly active, we're often seized by the powerful current of busyness, neglecting to question how best to utilise our valuable life on earth. People think, *"religion later, spirituality later, God later - first get on with life!"*

In Chapter Two we witness a role reversal. Arjuna seeks the counsel of Krishna, his chariot driver, who should be the one *receiving* orders. He inquires about his predicament, purpose, and how happiness can actually be found. Though surrounded by intensity, Arjuna makes time to recalibrate his vision. He resolves to *'Ask first, act later.'* In response, Krishna reveals something simple but profound - *"You are not this body,"* He says, *"but an eternal, indestructible spirit soul."* We're spiritual beings on a human journey! When our decisions factor in this crucial understanding, it re-routes our entire life trajectory, as Arjuna will himself experience.

Once, a group of friends visited New York and hired out the penthouse suite on the Hilton's 80th floor. They dropped off their bags and headed out for a bite of the Big Apple. After exploring the hot spots, they returned, exhausted and tired, only to find a sign on the hotel's ground floor which read *"Lifts out of order!"* Cursing and complaining, they reluctantly walked to the staircase, began their ascent, taking turns to tell each other stories to make it a little less painful. Having reached the 70th floor, they turned to one of their friends who had been unusually quiet and asked him to share something. *"My story is a complete tragedy"* he said. *"We're about to reach the 80th floor, but I forgot the room key at the reception desk!"*

People climb to the peak of academia, top the corporate ladder, reach the heights of social prestige, and then realise that despite all those 'successes' they forgot the key to happiness. To be happy, we must first realise who we are in the deepest spiritual sense, and then act in accordance with that knowledge. Curiosity sits within, and existential questions confront all of us at some point in life. The earlier we ask, the wiser we become, the more purposeful our lives will be. Einstein reminds us: *"Never stop questioning – curiosity has its own reason for existing."*

"Now I am confused about my duty and have lost all composure because of miserly weakness. In this condition I am asking You to tell me for certain what is best for me. Now I am Your disciple, and a soul surrendered unto You. Please instruct me."

(Bhagavad-gita 2.7)

References

2.7 – Human life is meant for inquiry into one's real purpose in life.

Living or Existing?

What is the difference between *living* and *existing*?

Contrast the two, reflecting on where you stand with regard to each indicator:

Existing	Living	Where I Stand
E.g. Seeking security	*E.g. Seeking discovery*	Existing
E.g. My life is controlled	*E.g. I control my life*	Mixed

Shifting Paradigms

Do you feel there is space for upgrading your life? What is your general trajectory - are you slipping more into 'existing,' moving progressively towards 'living,' or pretty much stagnant?

What causes us to 'exist' rather than 'live'?

What three things can you immediately do to make a shift from existing to living?

1.

2.

3.

3 spiritualists
DON'T AREN'T
owned

Spiritual and material are at polar opposites. The natural conclusion may then be that the spiritual journey veers away from the things of this world. People often think that spirituality requires one to give up affectionate relations, physical possessions and cherished aspirations. And even if it doesn't, they fear that the philosophising of spiritualists may cause them to lose all ambition in day-to-day affairs. As our spiritual interest grows, we often find that friends and family become visibly concerned – *"Don't become too spiritual,"* they opine *"otherwise you'll lose interest in life!"* Can we embrace the spiritual path and continue as functional, inspired and contributing members of society?

These confusions are carried not only by uninformed observers, but also by immature practitioners. Arjuna, who's in the process of digesting Krishna's words of wisdom, still has thoughts of leaving the battlefield, abandoning his worldly duties, and fully embracing his spiritual calling. He can't see the compatibility of pursuing a spiritual life and simultaneously honouring his day-to-day roles and responsibilities. To him, they're mutually exclusive.

In Chapter Three, entitled 'Karma-yoga,' Krishna expertly recalibrates Arjuna's vision. Real renunciation, Krishna says, is not in abstaining from the day-to-day world and distancing oneself from the 'material.' Rather, it's about giving up the greed, selfishness and envy that causes us to utilise 'material' things in self-centred and exploitative ways. The insightful wisdom of the Gita opens up the opportunity for someone to connect 'material' things to a higher spiritual purpose, and thereby utilise them in a way that brings spiritual progression. Everything in our life, be it our work, wealth, family or possessions can be integrally engaged as part of our spiritual growth. Those same things, when inappropriately used, bind us to misery; the house becomes like a prison, wealth becomes like chains, and all assets become a heavy burden weighing us down. Instead of owning things, we become owned *by* things.

An interesting anecdote about two monks offers a deep insight. Once, upon reaching a riverbank, they saw a beautiful lady who was stranded, unable to cross the knee-deep river. The younger monk ignored her and quickly paced across, cautious not to compromise his strict vows of celibacy. The older monk, however, politely went over to the distressed lady and offered a helping hand. She requested him to carry her across since she lacked the strength to contend with the river waves alone. Without hesitation, the old monk allowed her to climb his back, and he dutifully carried her over, after which they parted ways. The younger counterpart stood aghast, yet refrained from commenting. After hours of walking, still disturbed by the incident, the young monk broke his silence – *"How could you, a shining emblem of celibacy, carry a woman on your shoulders?"* he challenged. The older monk, hearing his immature estimation, looked straight back and replied – *"I carried that woman for a few minutes across the river for an essential purpose. You, my boy, have needlessly carried her in your mind for the last few hours!"* The message was loud and clear: real renunciation is within.

"Not by merely abstaining from work can one achieve freedom from reaction, nor by renunciation alone can one attain perfection."

(Bhagavad-gita 3.4)

References

3.1 – People mistakenly think of spiritual life as inertia or retirement from public life.

3.7 – One should function in the world and connect his activities to the spiritual cause.

Spiritualising

Identify two 'material' aspects of your life that can have an impact on your spiritual wellbeing. Examples could include relationships, responsibilities or facilities. Ask yourself:

What is this 'material' aspect? (*e.g. my marriage*)

What threat does this pose to my spiritual journey? (*e.g. time commitment and emotional involvement which reduces spiritual absorption*)

What would happen if I removed it completely from my life? (*e.g. feelings of loneliness and emotional vacuum*)

How can I redirect, harness or utilise it for spiritual benefit? (*e.g. do more spiritual activities together*)

Know

4

STUDY
through SINCERITY

So much of modern education is based around gathering facts, memorising information and regurgitating it in an exam. We're systematically trained to become repositories of data, bursting at the seams. *Does that really make one knowledgeable? Do formal certifications make us wise? Is knowledge meant to remain in one's head, or should it deeply transform some other aspect of our being?* When real education degenerates, we end up with more 'experts' but less wisdom – more information, but little transformation. This tendency can slip over into spirituality, where the study of ancient teachings becomes an academic pursuit and 'armchair' philosophy.

In Chapter Four, Krishna explores the topic of transcendental knowledge. As He ushers Arjuna onto the path of active spiritual life in this world, He highlights how transcendental knowledge guides that journey. Krishna explains the mechanism through which knowledge descends from a higher plane, what state of consciousness one must embody to receive it properly, and how humble interaction with spiritual teachers is absolutely necessary in order to grasp the essence. All of these points challenge our pride and vanity since they allude to the fact that our intellectual faculties, in and of themselves, are insufficient in making us truly knowledgeable. Transcendental knowledge is a gift that we receive - we can know it through what we become. Our own sincerity, demonstrated by a willingness to sacrifice and serve, as well as apply and share the knowledge with others, is the key that opens the treasure-house of wisdom.

Once, a man proudly declared, *"I can recite the Bhagavad-gita in 45 minutes."* Unimpressed, the guru replied: *"Can you live it for 45 minutes?"* That is the real challenge. When we take spiritual knowledge, deeply contemplate its meaning, conscientiously apply it in our life, and sincerely share it with others for their benefit, then the knowledge comes alive. The deeper secret of the Bhagavad-gita is that true knowledge is awakened in the heart by Krishna, who illuminates our consciousness when He is pleased by our selflessness and sincerity. True spiritual awakening is a result of grace.

A famous saint was once approached by an eager student: *"O master, O saintly person, you are in possession of many shining jewels of wisdom, carefully gathered from the ocean of scriptures. Can you give me those jewels of insight?"* The saint contemplated the young student's bold request and replied, *"If I give you those jewels freely you won't appreciate them, and if I sell you those jewels, you won't be able to afford them!"* Seeing the disappointment, the saint continued on, *"Instead, you must eagerly approach the sacred scriptures yourself. Study them with patience and humility, systematically navigating yourself to the depths, and there you'll discover incredible wisdom. Having grasped that wisdom, be sure to apply it to your life and bring the teachings into reality. Then, selflessly help others do the same. After doing this, look deep within your heart, and you'll find a treasure-house of resplendent jewels of insight."* It's not a cheap process.

"Just try to learn the truth by approaching a spiritual master. Inquire from him submissively and render service unto him. The self-realised souls can impart knowledge unto you because they have seen the truth."

(Bhagavad-gita 4.34)

References

4.33 – Key qualities required to understand the mystery of transcendental knowledge.

4.34 – Sincerity in approaching a spiritual teacher is absolutely vital.

Digesting Wisdom

Food enters the mouth, but only after chewing and digesting it can the nourishment be felt. In the same way, knowledge has its own process of digestion. There are four broad stages in spiritual learning:

1. **Hearing** (*sravanam*) – Receiving insight & inspiration *(Is it clear? What stands out? Do I have any questions?)*

2. **Reflecting** (*mananam*) – Deep contemplation & reflection *(What is my experience? What opportunities and difficulties does this bring?)*

3. **Applying** (*nididhyasanam*) – Practical realisation & application *(How does this relate to my life now? What changes could I make?)*

4. **Praying** (*vandanam*) - Heartfelt desire & supplication *(What prayer could I make in this regard?)*

Now consider the following passage and apply the four stages above to digest this wisdom in a deeper way:

"One has to approach a bona fide spiritual master to receive the knowledge. Such a spiritual master should be accepted in full surrender, and one should serve the spiritual master like a menial servant, without false prestige. Satisfaction of the self-realised spiritual master is the secret of advancement in spiritual life. Inquiries and submission constitute the proper combination for spiritual understanding. Unless there is submission and service, inquiries from the learned spiritual master will not be effective. One must be able to pass the test of the spiritual master, and when he sees the genuine desire of the disciple, he automatically blesses the disciple with genuine spiritual understanding." (Bhagavad-gita 4.34 Purport)

Sravanam

Mananam

Nididhyasanam

Vandanam

5
BE THE
TRY YOUR
Best

Couples are known to argue. In one such dispute, the disagreement became so acute that they had to settle it in court. There, they began arguing in front of the judge! The wife demanded, *"I want my son to become an accountant!"* while the husband countered, *"No! He should become a doctor!"* As it went back and forth, each side stubbornly defending their corner, the judge interjected and innocently asked, *"Why don't you just ask your son what he wants to be?"* The couple looked at the judge incredulously - *"our son isn't even born yet!"*

Each one of us are on the receiving end of our fair share of pressure and expectation. That powerful energy can inspire and elevate us, or depress and destroy us. Family, friends, society and the media set the bars of success, and we feel impelled to rise to the challenge. We want to be appreciated and accepted, acknowledged in a positive light, and we strive to make others proud of us. We shed blood, sweat and tears to create a life that looks good on the outside. Ironically, it may not feel very good on the inside. *Does our value lie in external achievements or something much deeper? How do we define real success?*

In Chapter Five, Krishna reassures Arjuna that far from impeding his spiritual journey, active life in the world can complement it. The key, however, is to function with detachment. Krishna explains that we cannot determine the results of our work, since there are influences which conspire beyond our control. Even when we try our best, things don't always transpire as planned. Though this may sound deflating, it's actually extremely liberating. We can only control our effort and endeavour - the rest is in the hands of providence. Knowing this, in times of achievement we feel immense gratitude, and in times of adversity we remain determined and hopeful, knowing that a higher plan is in place. Without this vision of spiritual dependency, our successes may cause us to become proud and complacent, while our adversities may bring loss of esteem and hopelessness, a feeling of being useless and inadequate. Success in life, Krishna says, is not to *be the best* but rather to *try our best*.

In the epic tale of Ramayana, we find a beautiful scene where herculean monkeys are throwing huge boulders into the sea, working to build a massive bridge so they can conquer the demon Ravana. There, we encounter one small squirrel. Some say it was contributing a few pebbles into the bridge-building exercise. Others say it was sliding dirt into the cracks to smoothen the jagged edges. One commentator mentions it was jumping into the sea, soaking up its fur with water, and coming back onto shore and shaking it off, hoping to dry up the ocean in that fashion! Whichever one it was, the monkeys were looking at the squirrel and thinking, *"Small! Insignificant! Make way for the heavy weight contributors!"* Lord Rama, however, was looking at the squirrel saying, *"Amazing! Wonderful! What a beautiful devotional offering!"* It's the wholehearted utilisation of our God-given capacity that counts. This is real success.

Putting undue pressure on ourselves to be high achievers may render us anxious, frustrated and even depressed. We can be ambitious, adventurous and bold, but must temper it with the deep spiritual awareness that our success is in *trying* our best. All subsequent results are sanctioned by Providence, beyond our circle of influence.

"The steadily devoted soul attains unadulterated peace because he offers the result of all activities to Me; whereas a person who is not in union with the Divine, who is greedy for the fruits of his labour, becomes entangled."

(Bhagavad-gita 5.12)

References

5.3 – Detachment from the results of activity.

Circles of Life

"God grant me the serenity to accept the things I cannot change, the courage to change the things I can, and the wisdom to know the difference." (Serenity Prayer)

In his book, 'The 7 Habits of Highly Effective People,' Stephen Covey distinguishes between our Circle of Concern and our Circle of Influence. The Circle of Concern includes the wide range of things that impact your life – health, family, finances, the economy, political situations etc. Your Circle of Influence encompasses the concerns that you can actually influence. For example, the state of the economy and climate change may concern you, but the average individual has little or no influence over them.

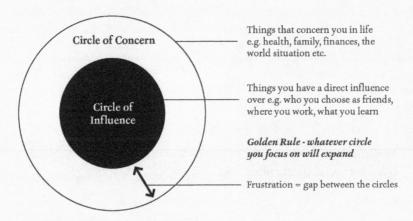

Circle of Concern

Things that concern you in life e.g. health, family, finances, the world situation etc.

Circle of Influence

Things you have a direct influence over e.g. who you choose as friends, where you work, what you learn

Golden Rule - whatever circle you focus on will expand

Frustration = gap between the circles

Progressive people focus their attention on the Circle of Influence. They identify what's in their control and put time, energy and resources into them. Here you can generate change, and when you do, the Circle of Influence grows.

Others become preoccupied with the Circle of Concern – the things over which they have little or no control. Because they focus on that which is (currently) unchangeable, they tend to become frustrated, and over time their Circle of Influence shrinks because they neglect it.

The gap between the two circles determines dissatisfaction and frustration in our life.

On a large sheet of paper draw these two circles and write down as many things as possible that sit within each one. Now reflect on how you are spending your time. Which circle are you primarily operating within?

Identify three things in your circle of concern that you unnecessarily focus on. How can you stop wasting that time and energy?

1.

2.

3.

Identify three things in your circle of influence that you are neglecting. How can you dedicate more time and energy to these things?

1.

2.

3.

train 6 your BODY MIND

How much money is spent on gym memberships? How much time is dedicated to grooming the body? How many elaborate plans are made to invigorate our physical vitality? Keeping the body fit, healthy and attractive is clearly a top priority for most people. While fixated on the external shell, however, we may have skipped a beat.

Take a look at your phone. The screen may be cracked, the battery knackered and the cover ripped, but you're still carrying it and the phone does its job. If the operating system crashes, however, the entire gadget becomes defunct; everything grinds to a halt. Attention to the invisible, intangible and subtle components of anything is absolutely essential. Thus, a wise person reflects on their life and asks – *"I'm maintaining the hardware of my existence, but what am I doing for the software of my existence?"* There's no point in a beautiful body minus a beautiful mind.

In Chapter Six, Krishna further explores identity and self-care. As spiritual beings, particles of consciousness, we possess two bodies, gross and subtle. The gross comprises of the visible physical frame, while the subtle consists of the invisible mind, intelligence and ego. The subtle body acts as an interface between the spirit and the gross. As spiritual beings, if we're able to appropriately harness the mind, it acts as a friend which supports and empowers us in the progressive journey of life. If not, the mind can deviate, discourage and damage us. From day-to-day, hour-to-hour and moment-to-moment, it can operate as the unseen enemy within.

Everyone can appreciate that we need steadiness of mind. When Arjuna, a consummate warrior of unparalleled strength, confesses that controlling the mind is more difficult than controlling the wind,

Krishna reassures him that it is indeed possible. How? By detachment (*vairagya*) and discipline (*abhyasa*).

First, we must learn to mind our mind; become an observer of the chatter. We shouldn't fall into the trap of identifying with every message that goes through our head. After all, the spirit soul is beyond the subtle and gross coverings. This vision of non-identification helps us utilise the positive, functional and empowering thoughts, leaving aside the negative, wasteful and destructive ones. Some thoughts, though tempting and exciting, divert us from our purpose. We shouldn't give up what we want most, for what feels good now. Through detachment, we learn to ignore many of the minds unwarranted demands.

Secondly, we need discipline. Former US President, Harry S. Truman, once said: *"In reading the lives of great men, I found that the first victory they won was over themselves. Self-discipline with all of them came first."* Detachment helps quieten the mind, and discipline then remoulds the mind. Krishna proposes daily spiritual practice with particular emphasis on early morning meditation. Such transformational practices can shift one's internal state if embraced with patience and perseverance. Though we naturally rebel against a regimen, that daily application is absolutely necessary. Otherwise we fall short of our potential. The pain of discipline is uncomfortable, but the pain of regret is unbearable.

"For him who has conquered the mind, the mind is the best of friends; but for one who has failed to do so, his mind will remain the greatest enemy."

(Bhagavad-gita 6.6)

References

6.34 – The characteristics of an uncontrolled mind.

Do Not Disturb

The mind is made of what? Thoughts. There are four broad types of thought – negative, positive, functional and wasteful.

Imagine your mind to be a room in which there are four different corners, corresponding to the four types of thoughts. In the room is a big ball of light representing your awareness. Whatever this ball of light illuminates will dominate your consciousness.

Reflect on your mind's activity yesterday and identify thoughts that came up under the various categories:

A Grid of Thoughts	
Functional	Positive
Wasteful	Negative

Mind control is all about empowering the functional and positive thoughts, and quietening the negative and wasteful thoughts. Engaging in spiritual practice and meditation are the most powerful tools we have to make this shift.

Please see the article in the appendix which details the spiritual practices recommended in the Bhagavad-gita. In this essay we detail the practice of bhakti-yoga and the various aspects that can be integrated into one's daily life.

HEAR to see to BELIEVE 7

Imagine a capacity-filled auditorium. As the show is about to commence, the MC steps onto stage, points at a random person in the front row, and asks: *"Can you tell me if Mark Naysmith is present in the audience?"* The unnerved audience member is noticeably baffled and unable to reply. It seems a simple enough question, but he remains unresponsive. *"Why don't you know?"* the MC challenges. Another uncomfortable silence. Innocently and nervously the audience member finally speaks out: *"Even if I could see everyone here, I still couldn't tell you, because I don't know who Mark Naysmith is!"*

Simple logic. If we don't know who God is, how He looks, what His qualities are, how He interacts with His creation, and what attracts His attention, how can we expect to find Him? The popular argument, *"First show me God and then I'll hear and study about Him,"* is inherently flawed. If we begin by hearing, studying and understanding God in depth and detail, then the prospect of finding Him becomes a distinct possibility. He may well be closer than we think, but without the necessary information, we'll be completely oblivious to the fact.

In Chapter Seven, Krishna guides Arjuna toward a greater revelation of the Absolute Truth. It all begins with deep assimilation of spiritual knowledge. At the onset of the Gita, we witness how Arjuna is seated right beside Krishna, and yet confused. As he hears the wisdom from Krishna's mouth, however, that confusion clears. Proximity to God, in and of itself, doesn't guarantee spiritual revelation – it is the patient, attentive and conscientious hearing of the message of God that yields one the desired benefit. People may be 'close' to God by dint of cultural upbringing and family tradition, but that alone does not trigger divine experience. The process of spiritual seeing begins through the ears.

Someone once referred to me as a 'man of faith.' I detected the condescending tone in his speech. It was, I'm pretty sure, a subtle put-down. Faith is often frowned upon in today's society – savvy people consider it unscientific, sentimental, primitive and a sign of weakness. Believe in what you see, they say, and take charge of fortune by shaping life on your own abilities and comprehension. It's a psychological approach originating from reductionist science, which aims to explain everything in mechanistic, empirical and routine terms. It's quite apt that the net result of 'reductionism' is to radically limit and impair our experience of life.

We can think of faith as trust – it is, without doubt, the most beautiful, extraordinary and empowering quality in existence! Without it, the world would be dull, dull, dull – life would be restricted to the tiny boundaries of our logic and rationale; pretty limited indeed. People say faith doesn't make sense, but that's exactly why it makes miracles. Someone believed there was something beyond the 'normal.' Someone knew there was a power and inspiration more profound than his own. Someone had the humility and wisdom to tap into a higher source of strength. Time and time again, we see how faith opens doors to the unknown.

Faith is the foundation of our spiritual life, and the Sanskrit word for it (*sraddha*) literally means *'to put your heart into something.'* As we deepen our faith through the process of hearing spiritual knowledge, an ordinary life morphs into a transcendental encounter with God.

"Now hear, O son of Prtha, how by practicing yoga in full consciousness of Me, with mind attached to Me, you can know Me in full, free from doubt."

(Bhagavad-gita 7.1)

References

7.1 – Hearing spiritual knowledge gives one the opportunity to connect with God.

7.2 – Complete knowledge requires one to accept a descending methodology.

Locating your Heart

Read the following statements and deeply consider what answer would fit most (if not all) of these statements:

You think about it all the time	
It drives your decisions	
You trust it to solve your problems	
You sacrifice all else for its sake	
You hold on to it as tight as you can	

Everyone will have their individual responses. A popular answer may be 'money.' Some people identify 'family,' or a special person in their life. Other people cite an achievement or accolade. Maybe it's a dream, a religion or a way of living?

Our answers are indicative of what we have faith in. Each of us put faith in something, and that naturally drives our decisions and life trajectory. The goal of the Bhagavad-gita is to help one nurture a relationship with Krishna, such that it becomes just as natural to put faith in Him as any of the things mentioned above. By investing in that relationship, crafting the connection through study, selfless service and spiritual practice, it eventually becomes completely natural to answer each one of these questions with 'Krishna.' That's the answer that won't let us down.

LIVE DIE before you Die⁸

Part of a monk's remit is to comfort the distressed. On one such occasion, we were driving to a funeral. We entered the crematorium gates, located the chapel, and parked in the first available bay. As the vehicle inched into place, we saw before us an ocean of gravestones. At that moment, almost prophetically, the satnav declared, *"You have reached your final destination."* Today the GPS was bringing home the truth!

Try as we may to avoid it, death is constantly knocking at our doorstep. Fast-forwarding a few years, we can anticipate that we'll grieve for loved ones, endure the devastation and emptiness of loss, and become personally weakened by the assault of old age and infirmity. All such experiences prepare us for our own inevitable exit. Despite this, we live in a society where death is sterilised, sanitised and carefully sealed off from public view. Statistics indicate that 72% of people die without writing a will. Maybe they thought it wouldn't happen to them, or perhaps they just didn't want to think about it. Despite our denial and defiance, time and tide wait for no man.

In Chapter Eight Krishna discusses this inconvenient truth. Most people focus on *living before dying*. They draw up a 'bucket list' of aspirations to pursue before time runs out - swim with the dolphins, visit the seven wonders, do a bungee jump and learn an exotic language. In our limited time on earth, people make plans to explore, discover, and experience as much as possible. *And why not?*

While there's no harm in excitement and adventure, Krishna reveals a deeper quest in the journey of life: to *die before we die*. To experience life in its truest beauty, we have to defeat the enemies within our own hearts - lust, anger, greed, envy, pride, and the multitude of material desires entrenched within us. Such qualities make our lives miserable, no matter how well the externals pan out. Furthermore, without this purification and cleansing, we'll be forced to re-enter the temporal realm after our final breath – to go through the trials and tribulations of the material world all over again.

Nelson Mandela was imprisoned for 27 years. Shortly after his release, when someone offered him a copy of the Bhagavad-gita, Mandela informed him that he had read it already. When asked what he learnt from his reading, the revolutionary politician smiled and replied: *"The Bhagavad-gita taught me that if I didn't overcome my bitterness, hatred and anger towards my perpetrators, though walking free from my cell, I'd still be very much imprisoned."*

We're held captive by the materialistic mindset and qualities present within our own being. To die before you die, means to break free of these invisible chains and live a life of freedom, here and beyond. The world needs more personalities who have embraced such saintliness. Nobody feels qualified, it won't be easy, and there will never be an ideal time. Along with all the dynamic plans to navigate the world around us, we could also consider the adventure of the 'inside job.' We say, we'll do it one day, although 'one day' is not a day of the week. 'One day,' Krishna reminds us, could be one day too late.

"Whatever state of being one remembers when he quits his body, O son of Kunti, that state he will attain without fail."

(Bhagavad-gita 8.6)

References

8.6 – What determines one's destination after death.

8.12 – Yoga withdraws one from materialistic entanglement, but how can that be achieved in today's climate?

Your Memorial

Sit in a quiet place, remove all distractions, and play some light, relaxing music. Now ask a friend to read the following passage to you.

Close your eyes, inhale deeply, withdraw your mind from the daily pressures and concentrate on the breathing sensation at your nostrils. Slowly take yourself on a guided meditation into the future.

Fast forward twenty years, and in your mind's eye picture a large gathering of people coming into a room. The mood is sombre and serious. You have departed the world, and this is the occasion of your own memorial service. Now try to picture the scene – Where have you gathered? Who has come? What are they thinking and feeling? How do you feel seeing them all?

Everyone is now seated and the person who knows you best comes forward to give a eulogy. Who would that person be? They begin to talk about your life, where you were born, your youth, education, where your first job was and your family situation. They talk about your interests and the major junctures in your lifetime. Try to envisage the speech.

Please turn over now...

As they begin to reveal their deeper feelings, how would you like them to complete the following sentences:

What I loved most about their personality was...	
Their greatest achievement was...	
They made a difference to the world by...	

When you reflect on your activities and character in the past week you can ask yourself what you have done to become the person that you have just described.

Krishna teaches Arjuna about his deeper identity, what the goal of life is, and where happiness is really to be found. Having this clarity at the beginning of each day helps us align our activities and energy accordingly. When we have clear answers to these questions that we have deliberated on, it helps overcome the external obstacles and internal blocks that may divert us from our real path in life.

This is an activity that can be done regularly in order to recalibrate your vision and reassess your priorities.

Give God wants
Ask for your what He
9

Janis Joplin famously sang, *"Oh Lord, won't you buy me a Mercedes Benz? My friends all drive Porsches, I must make amends. Worked hard all my lifetime, no help from my friends. So Lord, won't you buy me a Mercedes Benz?"* The world teaches us to approach God with a shopping list. A house by the sea, the latest HD screen TV, a multi-terabyte MP3...all about *"Me, me, me."* Is a divine connection meant for something more than just instantaneous health, wealth and prosperity? Can we really find satisfaction and love in such transactional dealings with the Supreme Person? What is the correct mind-set to approach God with?

In Chapter Nine, Krishna reveals a simple and sublime truth that most people miss. Nestled in the centre of this epic dialogue, Krishna imparts the most confidential knowledge. Though it's laudable to recognise God's supremacy and petition Him for our needs and wants, there is an alternative approach that brings deeper connection. Krishna explains how less intelligent people ask God for what they want, while the wise focus on giving God what He wants. That is love.

We can easily misuse the word 'love.' We say, *"I love,"* but what we really mean is *"I like."* There is a stark difference. Love is about giving, liking is about taking. Love is about serving, liking is about expecting. Love is about sacrifice, liking is about gratification. Once, a man was in a restaurant eating fish when a bystander walked over to him and asked, *"Is that fish you're eating?"* *"Yes"* the man replied, *"I love fish!"* The bystander didn't mince his words – *"No, you actually love yourself, and therefore you take the fish out of water, kill it, boil it and eat it! You* love *yourself... you* like *fish!"* A sobering thought. When a spiritual teacher was asked the difference between loving and liking, he pointed at a flower and said – *"If you like it, you'll go over to it, pick it, smell it and enjoy it. If you love it, you'll take care to water and protect it."*

The process of offering something with love is divine and mystical. Even when we feel we are lacking in love, when we focus on giving, serving and sacrificing in relationships, we'll find that love develops. When we give to someone, we're actually investing a part of our heart in them. When you give a part of your heart to someone, how can you not love them? Now you are a part of them! This love is known as *bhakti*, and when we direct this love towards the Supreme Person it's known as *bhakti-yoga*, the essence of the Bhagavad-gita.

Bhakti-yoga is not a ritualistic religious transaction, but rather a loving offering meant to reawaken a pure and intense love which lies dormant within us. While the process may appear simplistic and even mechanical, when practiced with sincerity and purity it actually combines and synthesises all other disciplines of yoga. Engaging in these practical acts of devotion will arouse the deep loving sentiment within each one of us, and direct it towards the Supreme Person who can most perfectly reciprocate with it. (*Please see the article in the appendix which details the spiritual practices recommended as part of bhakti-yoga*)

In this world people 'love' someone because they need them. That falls short of satisfying the heart. When we get to the point where we 'need' someone because we love them, then we'll experience what pure devotion is. Love is its own reward.

> ## "If one offers Me with love and devotion a leaf, a flower, fruit or water, I will accept it."
>
> (Bhagavad-gita 9.26)

References

9.24 – Seeking material benefit is unintelligent, but it can still bring spiritual elevation.

9.26 – Krishna is attracted by our love and devotion.

Daily Prayers

The majority of people in the world do make prayers, though what they usually pray for may not necessarily be so spiritual.

Write down three things you find yourself praying for regularly.

1.

2.

3.

Ask yourself:

If these prayers were answered would it actually make me happy?

If these prayers were answered what unintended consequences may I encounter?

How would I feel if someone came to me and repeatedly asked for these things?

Is there something more fundamental 'behind' these prayers that I am looking for? What is that, and will these prayers really fulfill that deeper desire that I have?

CAN'T see God ANYWHERE
CAN God EVERYWHERE

10

A teacher was lecturing. When she asked the children to repeat after her, *"I am an atheist,"* they all obediently followed. She did, however, notice a silent student at the back. When she asked him why he wasn't repeating, the young boy innocently replied that he wasn't an atheist, but rather a Christian. In a more challenging tone, the teacher asked why. The student replied: *"My mum is a Christian, my dad is a Christian, they taught me about Christianity, and now I am a Christian."* The teacher replied, *"That's not a very good argument - if your mum was lost, if your dad was lost, and if you were lost as a consequence, then what would you be?"* The boy paused for thought. *"Then,"* he said, *"I would be an atheist!"*

Some people can't see God anywhere. How incredible! The beautiful blue sky, the lively birds chirping, a carefree child chasing butterflies through a vibrant garden of blooming flowers, and the scorching rays of the dazzling sun. People marvel at nature's beauty, yet conclude it's all just random chemical reaction. They behold the deity of God and say, *"This is just matter."* They look at the Bhagavad-gita and say, *"This is just fictional."* They hear of people's spiritual experiences and say, *"That's just their imagination."* Despite the wonder of divine touch, they see only matter; they fail to detect the artist, the painter, the architect, the divinity behind the entire cosmos. They see but they don't see.

Having encouraged Arjuna to find a natural absorption in spiritual consciousness, in Chapter Ten Krishna goes on to explain how every sight of the world can trigger that awareness. Krishna says: *"I am the taste of water, the light of the sun and the moon, and the ability in man."* Whether it's that matchless experience of quenching our thirst with chilled water, the sheer brilliance of the luminaries in the sky, or the expertly gifted people that we encounter, we understand it all has its source in divinity. In a pure state of consciousness, the creation naturally reminds one of the creator, the design triggers thoughts of the designer and the artistry is an impetus to identify the artist.

In reality, however, we don't see things as they are, we see things as we are. What stands out in life is largely dependent upon the state of our own consciousness. Those who assimilate the teachings of Bhagavad-gita can see God everywhere, but those who don't may well struggle to find God anywhere.

But why isn't it blatantly obvious that God exists? How can masses of people miss the most crucial aspect of existence? Wouldn't such an astounding divine beauty shine out above and beyond everything else? Why is there even a shadow of doubt? It's actually an amazing exhibition of God's ingenuity to create the possibility of atheism. He designs the world in such a way that people can argue Him out of the equation! He leaves room for explanations that (at least externally) seem to coherently explain the universe in purely mechanistic terms. In other words, He doesn't make it a completely ludicrous proposition to not believe in Him. Since He wants a loving relationship, forged out of free will, He endows us with independence and offers an array of options. When we lovingly choose Him, we're able to interact face-to-face. That's the ultimate proof that we're all looking for.

"I am the source of all spiritual and material worlds. Everything emanates from Me. The wise who perfectly know this engage in My devotional service and worship Me with all their hearts."

(Bhagavad-gita 10.8)

References

10.17 – Even if one doesn't have a personal relationship with Krishna, He can still be seen through the physical world.

Missing the Obvious

See if you can decode the following statements using lateral thinking:

*1. It occurs once in an hour, once in a minute, but never in a second –
what is it?*

*2. A cat jumped out of a 30-storey building and lived – how is it
possible?*

3. What can you hold in your right hand, but not in your left?

*4. A girl who was just learning to drive went down a one-way street in
the wrong direction, but didn't break the law. How come?*

*5. There are six eggs in the basket. Six people each take one of the eggs.
How can it be that one egg is left in the basket?*

I won't give you the answers (you can check them up on the internet!) but if you're struggling, it's probably because you're not able to break free of a stereotyped way of thinking. In Question One people usually think about an event. In Question Two they make an assumption that's not stated. In Question Three they instinctively think of an object. In Question Four they draw up a picture in their mind and limit their thinking. In Question Five they get sucked into a default pattern of behaviour.

Krishna explains that the spiritual reality is free for everyone to access, but it requires clarity of consciousness. After hearing the answers to the questions above, we realise there is nothing esoteric at all – it's just simple and straightforward reality. Spirituality also becomes that natural when we're able to break free of our impaired and limited vision, which is based on assumptions and patterns of thinking that have been programmed into us over decades and lifetimes.

believe (11)
in YOURSELF KRISHNA

Modern self-development gurus teach us that confidence comes from within. You have to 'believe in yourself.' If you're sure, others will follow; *your* consciousness creates the reality. They tell us to be optimistic about our abilities, pride ourselves in our strengths, and have the conviction that anything is possible. This 'material confidence' may work in a limited scope for a finite time. Such confidence, however, which is rooted in artificial self-assurance, will inevitably dwindle, leading us to realise that we're not what we pumped ourselves up to be. In his prime, Muhammed Ali would proudly assert: *"I am the greatest."* Later in life he realised his folly, declaring that he was in actuality the greatest fool for attempting to usurp the Supreme position.

In Chapter Eleven, Arjuna discovers deeper truths about the cosmos. The most striking is the revelation that Krishna controls everything. Nothing moves without His sanction. *Uncomfortable or reassuring? Limiting or empowering? Depressing or hope-giving?* It all depends on how deeply we've understood ourselves, Krishna, and the relationship we have with Him.

In previous chapters, Krishna imparted His wisdom orally. Now, Krishna switches to a visual presentation. As He exhibits His Universal Form, Arjuna witnesses how past, present, future, and the entirety of existence rests within the Supreme Person. He sees how divine plans inevitably manifest according to the formidable movements of time. Arjuna realises that there are higher powers functioning way beyond his circle of influence. Struck with wonder and fear upon seeing the totality of creation and the imminent death of everyone on the battlefield, Arjuna requests Krishna to transform back into His unintimidating, original form. At that time, Krishna encourages

Arjuna, *"Conquer your enemies and enjoy a flourishing kingdom. They are already put to death by My arrangement, and you can be but an instrument in the fight."*

Arjuna's confidence is solidified. When we align ourselves with the divine will, transcendental back up is guaranteed. Real confidence comes from humility. We play our roles, fulfil our responsibilities, and endeavour with dedication, all the while knowing that we are acting on a stage which is being directed by higher powers. Despite our inherent limitations, we gain firm conviction from knowing that the all-powerful will of providence is on our side, which means anything is possible. One who is 'quietly confident,' their surety grounded in humility and dependence, can achieve unimaginable things in this world. Pride, complacency and hopelessness are not found in their dictionary. Seeing themselves as merely instruments, they sideline any ego or pride and let the divine magic manifest.

Despite having poor health, no money, no followers, and no specific strategy, Srila Prabhupada left India and came to the West to share Krishna Consciousness. His superpower was his unflinching faith in Krishna. Against all odds, despite innumerable trials and tribulations, he continued on with full faith. He became an instrument of spiritual inspiration, divinely empowered to spread Krishna Consciousness to every major city throughout the entire world. Not once did he take personal credit or glorify his own abilities. Rather, he always stressed that his dependence on divine grace is what triggered all the miracles.

"Therefore get up. Prepare to fight and win glory. Conquer your enemies and enjoy a flourishing kingdom. They are already put to death by My arrangement, and you, O Savyasaci, can be but an instrument in the fight."

(Bhagavad-gita 11.33)

References

11.33 – The entire creation is moving under the plan of God.

11.34 – The plans of God can be understood through His representatives.

Quietly Confident

It may seem that not being in control of your life is highly disempowering. Look at the table below, however, and consider how this profound truth may alter your approach to life and maximise your potential:

Situation	I control	Krishna controls
Success	Proud / Complacent	Grateful / Humble
Failure	Depressed / Frustrated	Accepting / Determined
Difficulties	Angry / Blame	Reflective / Progressive
Change	Nervous / Overwhelmed	Excited / Confident
Challenge	Inadequate / Weak	Empowered / Strong
Spiritual Journey	Hopeless / Unachievable	Hopeful / Achievable

Can you reflect on life examples for each of the above? For example, can you think of a time when you failed and became depressed due to your lack of spiritual awareness? Maybe you have witnessed someone who faced a challenging situation but became empowered due to their dependence on God? How can we develop the awareness that Krishna is in control?

make a list

12

TO-DO
TO-BE

Think of someone you truly admire. Now ask yourself – *"What is it that I appreciate in this person? Why are they so attractive?"* When we do this, one simple fact is highlighted again and again. We are drawn to people because of their qualities and personality. More impressive than their achievements and activities, is the character that such success is founded upon. People may acknowledge us for *what we do*, but they invariably remember us for *who we are*.

In an endlessly busy world, our focus is often on getting things done – having a 'to do' list. After all, that's what the world sees and that's what people applaud us for. Yet there is something more to consider. *What character have we cultivated? What qualities have we imbibed? What goodness do we exude?* When we die, people won't highlight the percentage we got in an exam, the position we were in the rankings or the number of people who followed us on Facebook. They definitely won't eulogise the price of our home, car, or clothes. The things that can be counted, don't always count; and the things that really count, can't always be counted.

Having shown the entirety of the cosmos to Arjuna, in the Gita's next instalment, Chapter Twelve, Krishna sheds some light on the inner world. He describes the charming character of an outstanding spiritualist which endears them to everyone. In our dealings with the Divine, the external offerings will never be that impressive... what unique gifts can infinitesimal beings really offer to the Supreme Creator? Yet, the purity of character and depth of devotion that a devotee exudes immediately attracts Divine attention, for Krishna is ever-interested in loving exchange based on pure selflessness.

Martin Luther King longed for the day when people *"Would not be judged by the colour of their skin, but by the content of their character."* In spiritual circles this is promoted. Alongside our 'to-do' lists which make us productive and efficient, we'd do well to create a 'to-be' list, reminding ourselves of the inner quality of our life and character. Thus, throughout the Bhagavad-gita, Krishna re-emphasises the qualities of highly successful spiritualists. He mentions tolerance, peacefulness, compassion, fearlessness, and forgiveness to name but a few.

It can be a struggle to imbibe such qualities in the practicality of daily life when situations seem to demand other responses. *Don't the peaceful have to be passionate at times? Don't the tolerant have to assert authority to resolve certain issues? Don't we all have to sometimes be fearful for the sake of survival?*

Such spiritual qualities are offered as a framework to guide our decisions, responses and wanderings in this complicated world. When deciding any course of action, the spiritualist remembers the cardinal principles they live by. However, one must have the wisdom to intelligently and appropriately apply such principles in any given situation. We may have a stereotyped image of how humble, tolerant and peaceful spiritualists conduct themselves, but these qualities go much deeper than the surface. The immediate acts we see with our eyes may not always reveal the true nature of someone's character; we have to appreciate the motivation and consciousness behind those acts.

"He by whom no one is put into difficulty and who is not disturbed by anyone, who is equipoised in happiness and distress, fear and anxiety, is very dear to Me."

(Bhagavad-gita 12.15)

References

12.13-20 – Qualities which endear one to Krishna and upgrade one's quality of life.

Practical Saintliness

One of the biggest challenges in developing spiritual character is learning how to appropriately balance the practical and the transcendental. We have to appropriately respond to real situations in the world, but we also have to live in a higher, almost other-worldly, state of mind. Embracing transcendence, but simultaneously down-to-earth.

Consider the following situations.

*1) You are walking down the street and you witness someone hurling racial abuse at an elderly man. How would **tolerance** be applied?*

*2) There is a huge natural disaster in Japan and you are asked to present a response in a public forum. How would **compassion** be applied?*

*3) You can see that someone is doing something self-destructive, but they probably won't accept any feedback from you. How would **truthfulness** be applied?*

Most individuals struggle to imbibe these qualities, while some endeavour to but without really helping the situation. A rare few manage to intelligently apply the quality in the most progressive way possible. How may one respond if:

a) They neglect the quality

1.

2.

3.

b) They superficially embrace the quality, but don't benefit the situation

1.

2.

3.

c) They intelligently imbibe the quality and progressively improve the situation

1.

2.

3.

Your 'To-Be' List: What are the five qualities that you would like to imbibe in your thoughts, words and actions?

1.

2.

3.

4.

5.

Display these five qualities in a prominent place and ensure you spend a few moments every day (ideally early in the morning) meditating on them.

God IS FAR IS NEAR seated IN HEAVEN WITHIN

13

Some traditions talk of a God who is far away in a remote realm. Even when you enter that spiritual abode, the interaction with Him seems sparse and somewhat formal. The 'distant God' resembles a fatherly personality who cares for us without being overly involved in day-to-day life. That God secures peace and comfort, somewhat of a cosmic order supplier; a convenient port of call in times of need and want. Not much extra is described about His personality, and even less about a personal and intimate exchange with Him.

In Chapter Thirteen, Krishna explains that He is closer than we may think. Seated in our hearts, Krishna is patiently waiting to guide the living being back to the spiritual world. There is the material body (*ksetra*) and the spirit soul within (*ksetra-jna*). Krishna, as the Supersoul (*paramatma*), accompanies the spirit soul through this temporary realm, waiting for the soul to acknowledge their relationship. The Supersoul is the overseer (*upadrasta*) and permitter (*anumanta*), and when the spirit soul turns to Him, He becomes enthusiastically active, making all arrangements to strengthen that relationship and navigate the journey back to the eternal realm.

Seated within, Krishna is indeed responsive. Sometimes, however, it feels as though God is very far away. In times of difficulty we especially feel that absence of God in our lives. We sometimes doubt that He is actually alive, alert and active. A seeming lack of reciprocation and intervention can discourage even the most dedicated spiritualist. *Where is God when you need Him? If He is so close why can't we see Him, even when we really want to? Does He really listen to our prayers?* Before answering those questions, consider the following:

Action – internal yearning should be accompanied by external endeavour. When the man made a diligent daily prayer to win the lottery, God was more than willing to acquiesce – if only he actually went out and bought a lottery ticket! Thus, it could also be that God wants to see a practical demonstration of our eagerness to see Him. What are we willing to sacrifice and what tangible efforts have we made to search Him out?

Reaction – we are not dealing with a cosmic order-supplier, but with a person. As persons, we don't mechanise our reciprocation, but rather respond on the basis of feelings and inspiration. Thus, one cannot force open the doors to see God, but can only humbly endeavour to connect with enthusiasm and determination. We should eagerly anticipate a divine audience, but simultaneously be willing to patiently wait.

Perception – maybe God has already intervened in our life, but not in the way we were expecting. Our ardent prayers are often accompanied by very specific expectations. When we carry stereotyped perceptions of how God should deal with us, we leave little room to witness how He is expertly working on a bigger and better plan that will satisfy our needs and desires in the deepest way imaginable.

"The Supreme Truth exists outside and inside of all living beings, the moving and the non-moving. Because He is subtle, He is beyond the power of the material senses to see or to know. Although far, far away, He is also near to all."

(Bhagavad-gita 13.16)

References

13.3 – Difference between the soul and Supersoul.

13.21 – Supersoul accompanies the individual soul through all chapters of life.

Answer my Prayer

Read the following poem, and try to recollect as many situations in your life which depict this:

The Blessings of Unanswered Prayers

I asked for strength that I might achieve; I was made weak that I might learn humbly to obey.

I asked for health that I might do greater things; I was given infirmity that I might do better things.

I asked for riches that I might be happy; I was given poverty that I might be wise.

I asked for power that I might have the praise of men; I was given weakness that I might feel the need of God.

I asked for all things that I might enjoy life; I was given life that I might enjoy all things.

I got nothing that I had asked for, but everything that I had hoped for.

Almost despite myself my unspoken prayers were answered;

I am, among all men, most richly blessed.

(Unknown Confederate soldier)

Meditation

Reflect on your life at present. With reference to scriptural writings and in consultation with spiritual friends, try to understand in what ways Krishna may be trying to bring you closer to Him.

the wealthy ⬤14

HAVE THE MOST NEED THE LEAST

Modern life is complicated – people have two cars, two houses, two phones and two television sets... is it all too much? As we rush around the world, we may well trade in our values for our 'valuables.' We strive to acquire and achieve – to create a life that looks good on the outside, but may not feel so good on the inside. Wealthy are those, the Bhagavad-gita says, who don't necessarily have the most, but who need the least. Internal satisfaction and contentment are the most prized possessions in the world.

Years ago people would walk or cycle from place to place. Then we advanced our civilisation and invented the car – convenient, quick and comfortable. The net result of this fast-paced lifestyle: at the end of a gruelling day at work, we drive that car to the gym, pay a monthly membership fee of £30, ride an exercise bike and pace on a treadmill, sweat our hearts out, and go absolutely nowhere! Stranger than this pattern of events is our unquestioning acceptance of it as 'normal.' It's worth stepping back and reflecting on the way we live. In our youth, we lose our health to gain wealth, then in our old age, we're forced to spend that wealth to regain our health. It's nothing short of crazy!

In Chapter Fourteen, Krishna presents a model of material reality that helps us recalibrate our desires, reflect upon our decisions, and reposition our eventual destiny. The environment, and everything within it, carries a certain influence – in principle, everything is tinged by goodness (*sattva*), passion (*rajas*) or ignorance (*tamas*). These are known as the three modes of material nature. The influence of goodness clarifies and pacifies. From it, qualities such as joy, wisdom, compassion and humility are born. Passion is said to confuse and provoke, giving rise to greed, anger, ambition and envy. Ignorance obscures and impedes, drawing one into laziness, delusion, indifference and idleness. The food we eat, the state of our environment, and the time of day, to name but a few, all carry the influence of the modes of nature. They all have an impact on our consciousness.

Krishna encourages us to engineer a lifestyle in the mode of goodness. This will help us maximise our potential, develop our character, and increase our overall sense of wellbeing and happiness. Since every decision builds our destiny, each one carries importance. Understanding the influence of the modes refines and empowers our decision-making, and facilitates a progressive destination in life.

Living in the mode of goodness can be summed up in the famous phrase coined by Srila Prabhupada - 'simple living, high thinking.' Individuals who embrace this ideal are rare. They strive for purity in a world of degradation, they embrace simplicity amongst rampant materialism, and they cultivate selflessness in an atmosphere charged with exploitation. Anyone who goes against the grain in such a bold way will undoubtedly be faced with temptation, doubt, ridicule and moments of weakness. This lifestyle and mindset in the mode of goodness, however, is the springboard from which one can develop their spiritual consciousness. In this consciousness, one experiences the happiness of the soul, incomparable to anything we may have encountered in this world.

"Material nature consists of three modes—goodness, passion and ignorance. When the eternal living entity comes in contact with nature, O mighty-armed Arjuna, he becomes conditioned by these modes."

(Bhagavad-gita 14.5)

References

14.12 - Dangers of mode of passion and an unbalanced lifestyle.

The Balancing Act

Go through the following questions and tick the ones you would answer 'yes' to:

Question	✓
1. I don't read spiritual books on a daily basis.	
2. I usually end each day with a huge list of things left to do.	
3. I feel uncomfortable and uneasy when I have time off and no pressing responsibilities.	
4. I regularly have a huge backlog of emails / people to contact / messages to answer.	
5. I feel like all my energy is taken up by work and career, leaving little energy for anything else.	
6. I feel my spiritual practices are mechanical.	
7. I consciously avoid spending time with others because I have too many things to do.	
8. I rarely reflect / introspect / scrutinize my life direction.	
9. I rarely do charity work or activities which are for the benefit of people I don't know.	
10. I find it hard to sleep / don't get enough sleep.	
11. I have lost a friendship over anger or failing to respect the other person.	
12. I rarely think about spirituality or question things around me from a spiritual point of view.	
13. When friends ring me I rarely have the time to have a friendly chat with them.	
14. I feel like I complain and find faults, more than being grateful and positive.	

Question	✓
15. I have health issues which are related to stress, anxiety, or irregular habits.	
16. I have not taken a holiday in a year.	
17. My partner or children sometimes complain that I don't have enough quality time for them.	
18. I don't have time to spend on self-development / exploring things I am interested in.	
19. If an emergency comes up in my life I find it very difficult to adjust.	
20. Most of my interactions with people are just about 'getting things done.'	

Evaluation

Count up how many of the statements were true for you. Here is the analysis:

0-7: Great! Keep going

8-14: Life Balance needs Adjustment

15-20: Danger! Urgent attention needed

Go back and look at all the statements you marked as true and consider what changes you could make to redress this.

pursue material dreams 15
discover spiritual reality

A travelling circus had arrived in town, and thousands flocked for a piece of the fun. The rule, however, was 'one in, one out' - only a single customer at a time. When the first lucky punter entered the blacked-out tent in anticipation, two wrestlers jumped out from nowhere and gave him a good lashing! He scrambled away, gasping for his life, exiting via the doorway he came through. There he saw all the eager faces waiting for their turn. *"How was it?"* they excitedly asked. He thought to himself: *"I queued up all day, paid good money to get in, and if I tell them it was miserable they'll think I'm a fool!"* He feigned a smile and bluffed - *"Brilliant show! You're in for a treat!"* The next person got the same beating and was faced with the same expectant crowd on his exit. *"How was it?"* they asked. He thought to himself: *"The last person had a great time, these people expected me to have a great time - I better tell them I had a great time."* And so he did. Like this, hundreds of people went into the circus, paid good money, had a terrible time, but all convinced each other it was wonderful. Fool's paradise!

Sound familiar? We're programmed to pursue material dreams in this temporary world - a successful career, the ideal family life, and an abundance of wealth, comfort and prestige. Following the trends, we're told to pump our time, energy and resources into living the dream. Most times we fall short of our dreams, and even when we realise them, the experience is not as exhilarating as we imagined. Often, we put on a façade to convince the world it's all going well. A projection of happiness; smiling faces, starving hearts. *Perhaps we're looking for the right thing, but in the wrong place?*

In Chapter Fifteen, Krishna compares the material world to an upside-down banyan tree. He describes how the real tree is the spiritual world, and the reflection in the water is the material world. In a reflection there is no substance, and therefore no satisfaction. Our expectations always exceed the reality, and we're left let-down and frustrated. Krishna coaches Arjuna to redirect his attention from ethereal dreams to eternal reality. All 'reality' outside of the spiritual world is ultimately a dream, and all 'dreams' in the spiritual world are tangible reality.

In the metaphysical realm, every step is a dance, every word is a song, every action is motivated by pure love, and the atmosphere is infused with ever-increasing transcendental happiness. Sounds good... maybe too good. Sceptics may posit that such ideas are embraced by escapists desperately seeking solace from the inevitable aches and pains of life. Krishna, however, describes this physical world as unreal – although it can be perceived by our human senses, it is constantly changing and has no endurance in the context of eternity. Far from the spiritual world being a distraction, the actuality is that the material, physical world is a distraction. To live in reality means to be fully conscious and aware of one's eternal identity, purpose and true home.

The soul has three intrinsic qualities - eternality (*sat*), sentience (*cit*) and bliss (*ananda*). When fairy tales tell us they 'lived happily ever after,' it's actually an expression of these innate qualities – lived (*cit*) happily (*ananda*) ever after (*sat*). To fulfil our most cherished, innermost dream, we have to reinstate ourselves in reality.

"The Supreme Personality of Godhead said: It is said that there is an imperishable banyan tree that has its roots upward and its branches down and whose leaves are the Vedic hymns. One who knows this tree is the knower of the Vedas."

(Bhagavad-gita 15.1)

References

15.1 – The material world is a perverted reflection of the spiritual world.

15.6 – The captivating beauty of the spiritual world.

Frustrated Happiness

When we search for happiness in material objects, experiences and relationships, our efforts will inevitably be foiled. The futility of material happiness plays out in four ways – can you think of examples in your life where you have experienced this?

Result of pursuing material dreams	Examples
Futility - Didn't get what you wanted	
Insubstantiality - Got it but didn't satisfy you	
Temporality - Satisfied you but didn't last / got bored	
Duality - Satisfied you but came with distress	

The pleasure derived from activities in the material sphere never really satisfies the yearning of the soul, forcing us to keep searching and seeking newer experiences.

Now think of spiritual endeavours. Why is it that sometimes one may feel the deficiencies of material happiness within their spiritual endeavours? Have you experienced a time when spiritual happiness was opposite to the above? What may we have to do in our life in order to consistently experience that spiritual happiness?

I, ME &16 MINE
WE, US OURS

A Rabbi was once asked to describe the difference between heaven and hell. By a wave of the hand he manifested a vision of hell; a group of hungry, emaciated men sitting at the dining table eagerly awaiting their lunch. The bowls of soup appeared. Problem was, their hands were in the shape of unusually long spoons – as they attempted to eat they just couldn't get the food into their mouth. It was agony! A veritable meal, but nobody could eat. The rabbi then waved his other arm and manifested a vision of heaven. Interestingly, it was the same dinner table, the same cuisine and the same long, spoon-shaped arms. In heaven, however, everyone seemed happy and healthy. As they began their meal, the secret was revealed. In heaven, everyone utilised their long spoons to feed the person opposite, and they were being fed in return. Perfect cooperation! The difference between heaven and hell: selflessness versus selfishness.

In Chapter Sixteen, Krishna distinguishes the divine from the demoniac. A demon is not necessarily a ghastly one-eyed creature with ferocious expressions and fiery weapons. They may well be walking among us, unassuming and unidentifiable, rooted in a way of living which distances them and others from spiritual progression towards the Supreme Person. There may well be a demon inside each one of us! In dialogue with Arjuna, Krishna clearly outlines the philosophy, mentality, activities and destiny of those with demoniac tendencies.

In the urban jungle, survival of the fittest is the name of the game. Our happiness is often founded upon the exploitation, mistreatment and detriment of others. If we are winning, it usually means someone else is losing. Spiritual communities of bygone ages, however, were based upon diametrically opposed ideals. Cooperation, respect and genuine concern for others were the cardinal principles underpinning social interaction. Sharing, after all, is caring. Wisdom teachers explain one way to decipher the degradation of society: first you'll have to purchase food, then you'll have to purchase water, and eventually you'll have to purchase air! Previously, these commodities were freely and lovingly exchanged amongst everyone. Nowadays people make a small fortune from selling them.

Selflessness even makes sense on a practical level. If every person in a community of 50 people is thinking about themselves, then everyone has one person looking after them. If each of us selflessly focus on others, then everyone has 49 caretakers! It may sound idealistic and utopian, but it really does work – for relationships, family units, organisations and entire communities. The depth and quality of any interaction is based on the degree of selflessness involved. Until we change the 'me' to the 'we,' genuine relationships, inner fulfilment and deep spiritual experiences will remain elusive. At every moment we're challenged to chip away at our own miserliness and become kind, open-hearted and generous souls.

To the degree that we live in the concept of 'I,' we experience illness. When we shift to the concept of 'we,' we'll experience wellness. The Gita encourages us to escape the small world of 'I, me, and mine,' and instead identify how we can sacrifice, serve, and bring happiness to others - in such gracious endeavours, our own happiness arises automatically. Mahatma Gandhi famously said, *"The best way to find yourself is to lose yourself in the service of others."*

"The demoniac person thinks: "So much wealth do I have today, and I will gain more according to my schemes. So much is mine now, and it will increase in the future, more and more."

(Bhagavad-gita 16.13)

References

16.12 – Demoniac Philosophy.

16.13-15 – Demoniac Mentality.

16.9 – Demoniac Activities.

16.19 – Demoniac Destiny.

Me to We

In order to truly awaken selflessness within the heart, we have to be convinced of its beauty and practicality. Reflect on the following questions:

Is it *Desirable*?

How would the quality of your life improve if you were more selfless? Wouldn't removing all selfishness make life bland and boring? Wouldn't we risk becoming bitter and frustrated if people don't reciprocate with our selflessness?

Is it *Practical*?

Can one who is selfless survive in this dog-eat-dog world? How would you avoid people taking advantage of you? Can you be selfless amongst materialistic people or is it something to cultivate amongst spiritualists?

Is it *Achievable*?

Is selflessness something that we can realistically expect to achieve in this lifetime? Have you seen examples of selfless spiritualists? What could be a practical way to advance towards selflessness? How do we measure our level of selflessness?

faith OPPOSES BUILDS **17**
knowledge

Investment of faith is a natural part of our psychology, and in cultured societies it grows organically. Unfortunately, regular exploitation and abuse of faith has promoted scepticism and suspicion as the orders of the day. Faith, they say, is for the weak and unintelligent. To live by your own judgement and discrimination is seen as rational and progressive. Yet even that's a farce, since everyone, regardless of their ontological standpoint, is impelled to put faith in something. When you fly across the world, you put faith in the pilot. When you pursue academic education, you put faith in an institution. When you navigate to a destination, you put faith in the GPS. Without faith, nobody can live. Without faith, we're rendered entirely dysfunctional.

In Chapter Seventeen, Krishna explains the divisions of faith. According to our mentality, we develop a certain type of faith. That faith moulds our lifestyle and endeavours, which thus determines the knowledge and experience we gain. Krishna invites Arjuna to develop a high-quality faith which will yield him a transcendental experience. Faith can bring one face-to-face with God. *How do we develop that faith and conviction? Are we required to begin with blind acceptance?*

Someone could propose that the true path to inner peace is to walk into your closest multi-storey car park and smash the windscreen of every blue vehicle while simultaneously screaming at the top of your voice! You could potentially do it, but I doubt anyone would. Aside from the small issue of criminal arrest, is the lack of any logical evidence to believe it's true.

While there are many options and choices in life, there is also an inbuilt screening process which filters out the nonsense. Amongst the many options in life, psychologists have explained that only 'live options' be taken seriously. A live option is *practical* – one can easily do it without any harmful consequence or drastic change to their life. A live option is *beneficial* – there is intrinsic value in it which makes logical sense. A live option is *probable* – many people have practically experienced the benefit of choosing it. If something is practical, beneficial and probable, it's obviously in our self-interest to seriously consider it. To whimsically reject such live options would be irrational, unintelligent and unjustifiable.

The proposition of the Bhagavad-gita is incredibly practical. It doesn't require massive lifestyle changes, but simple additions of yoga and meditation into one's daily routine. There are huge benefits on a physical, emotional and spiritual level that make logical sense and are directly perceivable. Further, millions of people testify to the profundity of the Bhagavad-gita, and gain immense spiritual wisdom, insight and inner peace from its teachings. While being cautious to avoid blind following, it would be just as absurd to blindly doubt something. To categorically dismiss the option, without any significant investigation, suggests a stubborn, irrational and illogical predisposition towards a certain worldview. How can one reject such 'live options' without thorough investigation, and simultaneously claim to be 'scientific' and free from subjective superstition?

"Anything done as sacrifice, charity or penance without faith in the Supreme, O son of Prtha, is impermanent. It is called asat and is useless both in this life and the next."

(Bhagavad-gita 17.28)

References

17.3 – Different types of faith found in people.

Building Faith

There are three crucial ways to develop your faith: Philosophy, People and Practice. Firstly, one should be intellectually convinced and have a strong 'why.' When we understand the purpose and logic behind what we're doing, we're much more likely to dedicate ourselves to it and remain unfazed in the face of inevitable obstacles. Secondly, one should surround themselves with inspiring spiritualists. The determination and faith of others is contagious and helps to carry us, especially when we are lagging behind. Finally, we have to dive in! When we practically reach out to connect with Krishna, we'll feel that personal reciprocation, which inspires us to reach out further.

Developing your faith is one of the most valuable investments you can make in your life. As is mentioned in the Christian tradition – *faith can move mountains*. Ask yourself:

	Activities to strengthen this aspect
Philosophy	
People	
Practice	

try

18
TO BE HAPPY
TO SERVE

Mothers are special. In an attempt to estimate the monetary value of 'motherly love,' researchers spent a week following one around. A typical day involved being a cabbie, cook, cleaner and counsellor to name but a few. They calculated the overtime the mother put in, and the unwavering dedication for years on end without any time off (even on family holidays she was fully on-call). After crunching the numbers, they discovered that to employ such a mother would set you back in the region of £100,000 a year!

That, however, doesn't tell you the full story; the quality of the job is what really stands out. The service of a mother is selfless and unceasing. They rarely stipulate any expectation in return for their services and jump at the opportunity to go beyond the call of duty. What to speak of receiving benefits, even when children act in dismissive and ungrateful ways, the mother happily continues to serve. Their sacrifice unfailingly continues day after day, and even when the child becomes a grown adult the outpouring of motherly love doesn't subside.

Ancient scriptures explain how our actions towards God and all living beings should emulate this quality of selflessness. By offering our lives in service, unmotivated and uninterrupted, we experience profound satisfaction and fulfilment which otherwise remains elusive. While this may be hard to conceive of, the living example of magnanimous mothers gives us an insight into what real selflessness looks like. Ask any mother and they know the satisfaction they feel. Srila Prabhupada explained how the love between mother and child is the purest form of love found in this world. How wonderful if we could take some moments to remember this, foster a mood of gratitude, and reproduce that selfless spirit in our spiritual endeavours. It would change our life, and it would surely change the world around us.

In the Gita's final chapter, Krishna brings home the essence of His teachings – it's service which awakens love, and love which satisfies the heart. The boy-saint, Prahlada, reveals a striking truth about happiness: *"One is happy as long as one does not endeavour for happiness; as soon as one begins his activities for happiness, his conditions of distress begin."* In our frantic attempts to find happiness we miss the whole point. Happiness comes from serving, from sacrificing, from selflessly giving. Pleasure derived from anything else will be fleeting at best. Krishna thus implores Arjuna to dedicate his life in selfless service.

It's interesting to think of a worldview where we are not the centre. *How can I not think about myself first?* It seems alien, unfulfilling and even scary. Ironically, that utter selflessness brings one to the most profound level of spirituality. Water the roots, and the whole tree automatically becomes satisfied. Feed the stomach and the entire body is nourished.

When our frantic search for selfish happiness stops, and we instead absorb ourselves in selfless service to God and His parts, we perfect our spirituality and experience true satisfaction of the soul. Nothing mystical, magical or esoteric about it: just the simple eagerness to serve. It's that simple. So simple, Srila Prabhupada once said, that we may just miss it.

"Because you are My very dear friend, I am speaking to you My supreme instruction, the most confidential knowledge of all. Hear this from Me, for it is for your benefit."

(Bhagavad-gita 18.64)

References

18.37-39 – Three types of happiness in this world.

18.55 – Devotional service brings one to the perfectional stage of life.

From Selfish to Selfless

We play various roles in our life, and each is an opportunity to embrace the mood of selfless service. Look at the table below and identify one behavioural change you could apply to become less selfish and more selfless in each of the roles you play.

Relationship	Less Selfish	More Selfless
With Spouse		
With Parents		
With Children		
With a Friend		
With Work Colleagues		
With Spiritualists		
With Guru		
With God		

Summary | Think Different

We can't change the world, but we can change the way we look at it. When we do that, the world looks completely different! By regularly contemplating these eighteen *sutras* and embedding them within your heart you'll discover clarity over confusion, opportunities over problems, and hope over frustration. Over and above everything, you'll see Krishna, face-to-face, and at that time everything will make perfect sense.

Are you ready to think different?

Part Two: *How to*

*The Bhagavad-gita transforms you
into the best version of yourself.*

	How to...
1	Become Determined
2	Make Good Choices
3	Overcome Temptation
4	Find your Purpose
5	Become Successful
6	Be Present
7	Avoid Mistakes
8	Face Death
9	Find Love
10	Perceive Beauty
11	Detect Divinity
12	Spiritually Progress
13	Find Freedom
14	Avoid Burnout
15	Become Detached
16	Change your Outlook
17	Perfect your Speech
18	Conquer Fear

Most people think of the Bhagavad-gita as a religious book. You can see why, but Krishna, the speaker, ironically concludes His teaching by recommending we abandon conventional religion, which can degenerate over time and become ritualistic, superficial and at best something cultural. Some people see the Bhagavad-gita as a philosophical book. That's true, and the Gita does indeed present paradigm-shifting insights which jolt us out of ingrained ways of thought. Yet there is more. Could we say the Bhagavad-gita is a spiritual book? That gets closer since many, regardless of religious or philosophical standpoint, are looking for a 'higher experience' of reality beyond the physical phenomena.

For me, however, the Bhagavad-gita is something far more universal and practical - a life companion. Religious or not, philosophical or not, spiritual or not, the Bhagavad-gita equips the reader with the vision and tools to navigate life, and its inevitable twists and turns, with grit and grace. All can benefit from its ever-fresh wisdom which empowers one to become the best version of themselves.

The Bhagavad-gita is the ultimate 'How-To' guide. If you're wondering how to make good choices, how to find success, how to be present in the moment or how to turn your life around, then look no further. The Gita doesn't simply encourage you to invest in a better after-life, but it empowers you to build a powerful *present life*. This ancient classic presents the quintessence of self-development.

Social media and the online world bursts with snappy and snazzy titbits of motivation that make perfect sense. We're reminded of the five cardinal principles of happy marriage, the three ways to diffuse anger, the four steps to enduring vitality, and the seven qualities that will win you the best friends on the planet; information meant to help us create a progressive, peaceful and pain-free life. Modern-day self-development promotes the ideals, but how much does it actually equip and empower one to genuinely imbibe this refined mental state?

A shift in our mindset and instinctive emotional response requires a deeper transformation of consciousness. There has to be profound existential awakening. Only when we see our life situation as a chapter of a longer story, when we understand that we are spiritual beings on a human journey, and when we deeply connect with the Divine Genius who is behind the workings of nature – only then can we function with genuine and sustained positivity. There can be no substantial self-development without spiritual development, since the self is by nature spiritual. To really improve ourselves, we must first deeply understand who we are and why we exist.

① how to become determined

Frank Clark, an American lawyer and politician, famously remarked that a path without obstacles is likely a path that doesn't lead anywhere significant. In spite of our well-intentioned plans, reality is peppered with unexpected blocks we may not have accounted for. The world is unpredictable to say the least, and in the face of adversity all kinds of doubts arise in the mind. *How many times have we begun something and given up?*

Unless the voice within says *"I want to! I can do! I know how to!"* the contrary voice telling us *"No can do"* starts gaining the upper hand. Ironically, many of life's failures were people who didn't realise how close they were to success when they gave up. A breakthrough may well be within reach but not always within sight. *How do we bolster our determination and avoid giving up too easily?* After all, the quality of our determination determines the quality of our life. We thrive on the hunger for a better future, and when we lack a vision, or lose the determination to follow the one we have, life becomes meaningless.

In Chapter One, Arjuna stands on the battlefield, his mind is reeling and the famous Gandiva bow slipping from his hand. In true warrior spirit, Arjuna had once made a vow to annihilate anyone who told him to leave aside his bow. To even think he would give up his fighting spirit was an insult. Ironic. This famed bow symbolises the determination of the living being to answer the call of duty and rise to the challenges of the day. The determination to heroically face whatever life throws one's way. The determination to never give up.

Just like Arjuna, many of us have, or will, experience a juncture in life where we're faced with existential confusion. We doubt our path and lose the will to continue. When we begin doubting our current identity and ideals, they begin to weigh us down rather than drive us forward. At that time we may opt to take a rest from them. It's interesting that the word 'depressed' is spoken phonetically as *deep rest.* When our life no longer inspires and excites us, we may well enter a state of deep rest and detach ourselves from everyone and everything. In Srila Prabhupada's translation of the Bhagavad-gita he explains that Arjuna's mind was in a state of depression. It's more common than we may think, and though there are acute forms of clinical depression, many more of us experience this in our own way.

In the seventeen chapters of dialogue that ensue, Krishna expertly equips Arjuna with a vision of life. When we have vision, then determination comes naturally. When we have a rock solid 'why,' we're willing to endure anything for it. The key is to find something which captures our imagination and resonates with our heart. Something which creates such a hunger that we're willing to do anything for it. Krishna shares with Arjuna the greatest vision, goal and adventure that anyone could embark upon – the journey within. In life, we often set a plethora of external goals to aim for, but overlook the inner adventure. When the immensity of this spiritual quest, the journey of self-discovery, dawns on us, it subsumes all difficulties and generates an unbreakable determination. Equipped with spiritual vision, nothing can faze you.

"Sanjaya said: Arjuna, having thus spoken on the battlefield, cast aside his bow and arrows and sat down on the chariot, his mind overwhelmed with grief."

(Bhagavad-gita 1.46)

References

1.21-22 – At the onset of war, Arjuna begins to reassess his mission and priorities in life.

My Mission

Reflect on the following sentences and complete them with honesty and authenticity:

I thrive in life when	
I lose my drive and motivation when	
I am truly happy when	
I want to be a person who	
Someday I would like to	
My greatest talents and strengths are	
For me, the most important thing in life is	

Writing a Statement

The process of writing a personal mission statement requires deep reflection about who we are and what our purpose is. It is something that will require many attempts, and will inevitably evolve over time. Once you have a draft, mark yourself out of 10 on whether this mission statement ...

- Challenges and motivates you
- Encapsulates your vision and values
- Establishes your roles and responsibilities in life
- Identifies something tangible and measurable
- Represents the unique contribution you can make

Now go back to your statement and address the aspects which are weak.

② how to make decisions

Scientists say we make up to 35,000 decisions every single day. Some are practical – when we'll get up, what we'll wear and how we'll fit everything into the day. Other decisions are more tactical and strategic – where we'll live and what we'll study. As the world becomes increasingly complex, the options available expand exponentially, and people begin suffering from decision-making fatigue. Life can seem like a perpetual multiple-choice exam, and making those decisions is not always easy. It can be disconcerting, since decisions determine destiny.

There are three broad archetypes in decision-making. Some of us are just *indecisive*. We struggle to commit, perpetually sitting on the fence, unwilling to take a stand and assertively embrace a clear path. On the polar opposite are the *impulsive*, who dive in and decide without scrutiny and due diligence. The *introspective* decision-makers walk the middle path. They embrace the opportunity of choice, but carefully investigate and contemplate the likely ramifications of each option. Interestingly, the Bhagavad-gita opens up a fourth dimension in decision-making which is relatively untapped, but which can be a complete game-changer.

Arjuna was sweating. With deafening conchshells sounding, the armies gearing themselves up, and the weight of expectation on his shoulders, the atmosphere had well and truly reached fever pitch. He was baffled. How to honour his various responsibilities, preserve his morality, and decipher a course of action that would please everyone? He was trying to avoid indecision and impulsiveness, and thus came to the middle of the battlefield and began an introspective analysis. The game-changer, however, occurred when Arjuna, in order to upgrade his introspection, added the element of *inspiration*. That elevated source of insight, beyond the limits of our own mind and intelligence, opens the doors to enlightened decision-making.

Arjuna's inspiration was Krishna, an endless fountain of knowledge and wisdom who knew the answers, and was able to convey them in a digestible and practical way. We all need perspective in our life – rising to a vantage point beyond our own limited vision reveals the bigger picture. How we wish we could turn to Krishna whenever a decision-making dilemma arises. Arjuna was exceedingly fortunate, but where do *we* find our inspiration?

To be inspired etymologically means to 'infuse with a spirit,' and usually indicates some form of divine guidance. According to spiritual tradition, this divine guidance is available to us in the here and now, almost at our fingertips. Firstly, there are the divine books, which are not just historical writings but a living theology, fully equipped to address one's confusions and concerns. Then there are the divine guides, spiritually inspired individuals who can expertly administer the wisdom in a tailor-made way. Finally, there is the Supersoul, the divinity within, the voice of intuition that injects surety and conviction. The depth of one's connection with these three sources of spiritual inspiration will directly impact the quality of one's decision making. Despite his initial bewilderment, Arjuna went on to make the most powerful and pertinent decisions of his life. It was all possible due to the very first decision he made – the decision to take inspiration from a higher source. That was indeed the game-changer.

"Nor do we know which is better—conquering them or being conquered by them. If we killed the sons of Dhritarastra, we should not care to live. Yet they are now standing before us on the battlefield."

(Bhagavad-gita 2.6)

References

2.7 – Arjuna admits that he requires help and is unable to independently find a solution.

2.8 – No amount of speculation, however qualified one may be, will bring one definitive answers.

Decisions Decisions

Think of the three biggest decisions you have made in your life, and then rate yourself out of 10 on each one (10 being a very good decision, 1 being very bad).

1.

2.

3.

Now look at the weakest of those decisions and ask yourself:

What were the positives and negatives of the decision-making process you took in that instance?

Positives	Negatives

If you were to take that decision again how would you incorporate more introspection and inspiration?

In general, what are your weak points in decision-making and what can you do to change that?

Managing Emotions

In decision-making, one of the biggest challenges is that the emotions we are feeling in that moment override our good intelligence. Can you think of bad decisions you made when you were experiencing the following emotions:

a) Angry b) Excited c) Desirous d) Fear e) Grief

What can you do when emotions are running high, so you don't end up making a decision that you later regret?

3 how to overcome
temptation

It's so easy to trade in what we want most for what feels good now, seemingly impelled to act against our better judgement time and time again. For example, the cautionary messages on cigarette packets have intensified over time, yet the demand hasn't diminished. First the caution read '*Smoking may damage your health,*' and later it was more strongly edited to '*Tobacco causes cancer.*' To further highlight the dangers they alerted people that '*Smoking kills,*' and nowadays they've added shocking pictures of what goes haywire inside your body. Amplified messages, falling on deaf ears. *How do we break free of temptation?*

In the previous chapter, Krishna upgraded Arjuna's intelligence with paradigm-shifting insights that transform our vision of life. Yet Arjuna is streetwise and he knows the down-to-earth challenge of what it means to try and live this in real life. We may be intellectually convinced, but having the internal strength to follow it through is a different ball game. His question: "*Even when we know the right thing, why is it that we often act against our own will, as if impelled by force?*"

In Chapter Three, Krishna exposes the hidden enemy of every single struggling soul in this world – lust! When we are infected by this strong urge of selfishness and 'me-centred' mentality we do irrational and unthinkable things to satisfy our desires, even when it causes harm to ourselves and others, and diverts us from what we seek most. As Oscar Wilde once said: "*I can resist everything except temptation!*"

Someone once asked me: "*If God wants us to do the right things, why does He give so many wrong options?!*" I responded that in multiple choice exams there are always more wrong answers than right. If you approach those exams unprepared then the odds are always stacked against you. If you've familiarised yourself with the lessons, however, those exams are a walk in the park – the right answer just jumps out! Yes, there may be so many diversions in this world, but even small doses of spiritual knowledge go a long way in helping us identify what path to tread.

Since the enemy of lust has captured strategic points, we have to be aware, equipped and ready for combat. The scriptures give four major hints to overthrow the enemy and emerge victorious:

Conviction (intellectual space) – believe in your aspiration, and understand why discipline and self-restraint are essential. That clarity of purpose creates an inner strength.

Openness (emotional space) – regardless of success or failure, be open with a friend and seek advice, support, guidance and feedback. There is no purity without honesty.

Safety (sensual space) – avoid provoking situations, interactions and lifestyles that may compromise your principles. Stay away from temptation, and don't fight unnecessary battles.

Taste (spiritual space) – strive to create the 'better life,' and solidify your resolve by tangibly experiencing the benefits of your restraint. Invest in forging a divine connection, something pure and uplifting which will yield a 'higher taste.'

"Arjuna said: O descendant of Vrsni, by what is one impelled to sinful acts, even unwillingly, as if engaged by force?"

(Bhagavad-gita 3.36)

References

3.37 – Krishna identifies lust as the all-devouring enemy.

3.38 – Every living entity is covered by different degrees of lust.

A Battle Plan

Think of an area of your life where you are regularly falling prey to temptation and destructive behaviours.

Write down the emotions / feelings that you have when you fall victim to this.

Now make a plan which will help you to develop the strength and resolve to resist this:

Conviction – have a strong why:

Write down a) how your life would improve if you were able to refrain from this b) examples of real-life success stories in this regard c) glimpses of this success that you have witnessed in your life

Openness - have a good friend:

Write down a) what benefit could come if you share your struggles / successes with someone else b) what stops you from being open with someone c) who is a person that you could confide in

Safety - have the right surrounding:

Write down a) situations, interactions, mindsets which make you vulnerable to this weakness b) practical changes you could make to strengthen your resolve c) new environments you could create which would bring positive energy

Taste - have a sense of inspiration:

Write down a) situations where this weakness has disappeared due to engagement in something more progressive b) activities which bring you inspiration and strength c) spiritual engagements you need to invest in

how to find
purp⁴ose

Have you ever looked back at your life and questioned what you've achieved? Many feel unproductive and unenthused, not sure what they should be doing and where they'll make a difference. In moments of doubt we usually shrug it off and return to the daily grind. We surrender to the fact that life is what it is, and amidst responsibilities, expectations and daily demands we resign ourselves to the life we have created, never really addressing our inner calling. Ironically, it's that inner calling which is the essence of our being – our unique gifted individuality that brings forth our special contribution to the world. If we ignore that, we disregard something valuable we've been invested with.

We could be compared to mobile phones, each one with ingenious apps, unique features, and savvy specialities. Some are lighter, some are more durable, and some have a battery power that outlives other models. Regardless of the variety, each and every phone has the capacity to perform the most fundamental task – to call and connect with someone.

In the same way, we each have unique abilities, strengths, personalities and capacities inbuilt within our body and mind. When we identify and engage these, we embrace our *sva-dharma* – occupational duties that we are 'wired' for in this life. Beyond the body and mind, as spiritual beings, we each have a *sanatana-dharma* – the essential and eternal function of connecting with the Supreme Person, the most fundamental aspiration within each one of us. The Bhagavad-gita teaches how to embrace our purpose, our *dharma*, on the immediate and ultimate level.

Thus far, Krishna has consistently advised Arjuna to remain in the active world. In Chapter Four, He helps Arjuna to identify the most effective and efficient way to function. There are four broad categories of *dharmic* engagement, and Krishna reassures Arjuna that he is correctly situated as a warrior. This framework, known as *varnasrama*, is a powerful reference point to identify our unique *dharma*. Happy and fulfilled people utilise wisdom and guidance to accurately understand what makes them tick. It's a simple but neglected principle of life. We live in a noisy world, and, in the midst of it, struggle to pinpoint our calling. If we don't, we'll find daily duties are slow and tiring, require excessive effort and attention, feel uncomfortable and abnormal, and fail to harness our innate potential. We're left feeling unfulfilled and unhappy.

The problem can, however, go beyond this. It's difficult to *find* your *dharma*, but just as challenging to wholeheartedly *live* your *dharma*. Even when we know what we are 'hard-wired' for, various factors deviate us from the path we should be treading. The expectations of others, the desire for appreciation and accolade, the restlessness and intrigue of trying new things, and the common delusion that the grass is greener on the other side. These are all factors which lure us towards the unnatural and set us up for disappointment and failure. Honest living is about doing what you are truly meant for, however big or small, in whatever field or arena, regardless of pressure or public opinion. Everyone, without exception, has something unique to bring to the table. We only have to find it and feed it.

"According to the three modes of material nature and the work associated with them, the four divisions of human society are created by Me. And although I am the creator of this system, you should know that I am yet the nondoer, being unchangeable."

(Bhagavad-gita 4.13)

Finding Purpose

In the Bhagavad-gita, Krishna identifies four broad categories of social contribution. See the table below and reflect on your strengths and aspirations, and try to identify what role is most fulfilling to you. :

	Brahmana (Educator)	Ksatriya (Executive)	Vaisya (Entrepeneur)	Sudra (Employee)
Activity	Teach	Manage	Supply	Assist
Value added	Knowledge	Protection	Wealth	Stability
Fights	Ignorance	Injustice	Insufficiency	Indolence
Qualities	Self-control, austerity, purity	Heroism, power, fortitude	Farming, cow protection, business	Simplicity, loyalty

Based on this information, try to ascertain your ideal occupation. Here are three tips to help:

Analyse – reflect on your qualities and character, and conduct a personality test. Try to identify the things you are good at, and those things you are attracted to. The intersection between these two aspects certainly indicates integral parts of your *dharma*.

Ask – draw upon the advice of friends, mentors and coaches. We can't always analyse ourselves in an objective way, but neutral (and informed) observers can offer greater clarity.

Attempt – try different things, experiment and don't be afraid to fail. Even when we attempt something and find it's unsuitable, it helps us to decipher what may well be suitable. We should embrace the growth and wisdom that comes with failure.

5 how to become successful

The ancient texts outline some broad indicators of *karmic* merit – respectable birth, abundance of wealth, sharp intelligence and good looks. According to our activities in previous lives, we are rewarded with a specific configuration of these. In this life, most people work hard to enhance and upgrade what they have – we attempt to climb the social ladder, expand our riches, educate ourselves to intellectually outshine others, and beautify the body as far as possible. People invest unspeakable amounts of energy into such endeavours.

Continuing the theme of remaining in the world, Krishna shares an essential paradigm to etch within our being. In Chapter Five He explains that we're not entirely in control of success or failure in our material endeavours, but rather there are factors beyond us that are influencing the outcome. The expected rewards may or may not appear, and regardless, we shouldn't become too fixated on them, because even when they do appear, they don't actually bring happiness.

Most of us, however, are convinced we are in control. Thus, when we fail to achieve certain goals we feel deflated. In success we're also dissatisfied because we quickly realise that the vacancy within the heart remains. The famed Queen Kunti states that only when we retire from the rush for these ephemeral rewards, can we really and truly embrace the spiritual path. When we invest our hopes and energies in material success, not only do we internally starve, but we're overcome by the three cancers of the mind - comparison, competition and criticism. Perpetually dissatisfied because enough is never enough.

Some years ago, 'The Secret' by Rhonda Byrne, was a book everyone was reading. The secret that Byrne felt she had discovered was the 'law of attraction': whatever you think about and focus on, eventually becomes your reality. The universe, she said, is essentially energy, and all energy vibrates at different frequencies. Since each person also vibrates at a certain frequency, they attract the same within the larger energy field. Thus, we attract objects, fortunes, people and situations that are of a similar 'vibration' to ourselves.

It's a mouth-watering concept – the possibility of attracting anything you desire. While the Bhagavad-gita would agree with the general notion of designing our destiny, there is more to the story. Philosophical exploration and practical observation clearly reveals that we are not the sole dictators of our fortunes. There's something called *karma*. We may desire a variety of things, but without the necessary karmic credit, those things will remain elusive. The secret, then, is not as simple and straightforward as it sounds.

The Bhagavad-gita, however, reveals a more profound secret to life. While Rhonda's book is about attracting, the Gita encourages one to first establish what is worthy of being attracted. Most people hastily draw up their shopping lists of life without significantly considering this point. Our basic problem is that we're attracted to the wrong things - things that won't bring us what we're ultimately looking for. When we redefine success, turn our attention towards the right things, spiritual things, things that allow us to connect with our very essence, then everything falls into place perfectly. This is the secret behind the secret.

"One who works in devotion, who is a pure soul, and who controls his mind and senses is dear to everyone, and everyone is dear to him. Though always working, such a man is never entangled."

(Bhagavad-gita 5.7)

References

5.12 – The art of how to live and work like a lotus, untouched by the water.

5.14-15 – The three doers - the living entity desires, the Supreme Lord sanctions and material nature facilitates.

Building Blocks of Success

Think of three successful people who have achieved something great in the world, spiritually or materially. For these individuals please fill out the following table:

Who?	What did they achieve?	What qualities were behind it?	How could I apply that quality in my life?	What stops me from applying that quality?

When you see the achievements of others, try to delve a little deeper and see what is behind it. Focusing solely on their achievements will not lend us the information and inspiration required to empower our own life. We can learn from everyone but must realise we are on our own journey.

how to be
present

Have you ever watched a movie that's out-of-sync? When the audio and video are misaligned it's practically impossible to give your full attention – the lack of congruence is too annoying! Our life can often become like a dubbed, out-of-sync film; the body in one place, but the thoughts in quite another. Such absent-mindedness impairs our capacity to appreciate life and achieve our highest potential.

The mind has become one of the biggest talking points in 21st Century medicine. Never before have we had such surging numbers of people experiencing issues in their psychological space. Though unnatural lifestyles and imbalanced habits have clearly contributed to it, the problem of the mind has been a perennial one, whether or not we define it in today's clinical terms. Thus, a significant amount of dialogue in the Bhagavad-gita is dedicated to the subject of the mind – how to identify it, understand it, control it and ultimately harness it for wellbeing and spiritual elevation.

In Chapter Six, Krishna highlights that control of the mind and the ability to bring it to the present moment is an integral aspect of all *yoga* practice. Without reforming the useless, distracting and annoying mental chatter, we can't really progress. The mind travels and absorbs – it enters into objects, places and people, and they can easily enter into it! The mind has a dreamy tendency to assume things were better in the past or they'll improve in the future, unwilling to wholeheartedly embrace the situation as it stands. It often sees the problems in every opportunity, instead of seeing the opportunities in every problem. The mind, it seems, is on a relentless mission to distract us from finding perfection in the present.

It's not that the past and future are irrelevant. We have to learn from what has happened, and surely we plan for what may come. Yet in the midst of that we have to find a way to live in the moment. Many, however, have resigned themselves to the mental state they find themselves in, convinced that there is no way to reform the uncontrolled mind and escape the negativity and limiting thoughts that subsume them. Krishna, however, offers multiple tools to remould the mind, most powerful of which is *mantra* meditation.

The metaphor of an internet browser can help us understand the mind. Just as Mozilla Firefox has a default homepage, the browser of our mind has a default fall back – a vision and way of thinking that it always returns to. We have favourites in our browser, and the mind similarly entertains desires and dreams that have been inspired by people and places. Just as a browser has a history, the mind is ingrained with impressions from past experiences. A browser has an autocomplete, offering options according to where we've browsed before. The mind also gravitates towards experiences and emotions which immediately resonate.

Thankfully browsers can be reconfigured; browsing data deleted, settings personalised, aesthetics adjusted and updates installed. The mind is no different. Step by step, bit by bit, slowly but surely, we can craft a beautiful mind that walks with us in the here and now. Beware, however, because even optimised browsers are subject to pop-ups! While we live with this mind, there will always be that inescapable element of unpredictability. Fear not, however, the trick is to identify the mind, instead of identifying *with* the mind!

"Lord Sri Krishna said: O mighty-armed son of Kunti, it is undoubtedly very difficult to curb the restless mind, but it is possible by suitable practice and by detachment."

(Bhagavad-gita 6.35)

References

6.35 – Control of the mind can be achieved through practice and detachment.

Mantra – Free the Mind

For some, the repeated recitation of God's names may seem a mechanical and somewhat elementary spiritual practice. How can the utterance of mere sounds - linguistic formulations - transform consciousness and invoke spiritual experience?

The holy name of Krishna has extraordinary spiritual potency because the name of God is non-different to God Himself. Language, in the material sense, is merely representative and symbolic; it does not itself embody the reality it seeks to represent. God, on the other hand, is absolute, and thus there is no difference between Him and His name. When one chants the names of God with pure intention and dedicated attention, they actually come in direct contact with Him. In the Absolute realm, symbol embodies reality.

Hare Krishna Hare Krishna Krishna Krishna Hare Hare
Hare Rama Hare Rama Rama Rama Hare Hare

Chanting the *Hare Krishna mantra* is considered the most important activity for spiritual and mental wellbeing. The *mantra* essentially a prayer that means *"O energy of the Lord (Hare), O all-attractive Lord (Krishna), O supreme enjoyer (Rama), please engage me in Your service."*

Chanting as a personal meditation is known as *japa*. The best time for *japa* is the early morning since the atmosphere is quiet and the mind is not yet preoccupied with the activities of the day. If that's not possible, set aside another suitable time slot in the day. *Japa* meditation is best performed on beads, which assist us in counting the *mantras* and keeping good concentration.

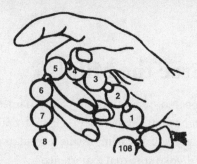

Hold the beads in your right hand, between the thumb and middle finger. Begin chanting after the big centre bead (which is known as the 'Krishna bead') (see diagram)

Chant the *mantra* softly but distinctly, pronouncing it in such a way that you can hear it clearly.

Then move onto the next bead, and repeat the mantra.

By the time you get back to the Krishna bead, you will have chanted the *Hare Krishna mantra* 108 times. This is called one 'round'.

Then turn the beads around and start the second round without crossing over the Krishna bead

In the beginning, one round may take you fifteen minutes or so but as you get used to chanting you will usually speed up to between six and eight minutes. You can begin with one round a day and gradually increase. Once you commit to chanting a certain number of rounds daily, try not to go below this number. It's far better to chant two rounds every day than eight rounds one day and none the next. Consistency is essential for our spiritual progress.

The main principle of chanting is to attentively listen to the sound vibration. The *mantra* is chanted by the tongue and immediately caught by the ear. If any distracting thoughts come into your mind, bring your focus back to the sound of the Hare Krishna *mantra* and those thoughts will eventually disappear. In this way, our original spiritual consciousness is gradually reawakened.

⑦ how to avoid
mistakes

One of the major branches of philosophy is epistemology – the theory of knowledge, or plainly put, how you know what you know. Jiva Goswami, one of the greatest philosophers of all time, identified various *pramanas*, or sources of knowledge. Broadly speaking, there are three – *pratyaksa, anumana* and *sabda. Pratyaksa* refers to knowledge gained from one's sensual perception, while *anumana* refers to that which is concluded via inference of the mind. *Sabda* is knowledge which is faithfully received from an external source.

Humans, Jiva Goswami says, are inherent with four defects. To begin with they have imperfect senses, and thus are susceptible to falling into illusion. Because of this, they're prone to making mistakes, and this often incites the propensity to cheat in order to cover it all up! Any introspective person can observe this pattern of behaviour. For this reason, *pratyaksa* and *anumana*, which rely on our limited sensual and mental faculties, are inherently flawed – anything sourced from them cannot be foolproof. If one employs *sabda-pramana*, but receives knowledge from another human being, they find themselves in the same predicament. Jiva Goswami's conclusion: to gain perfect knowledge one must employ *sabda-pramana* by hearing from a *non-material* source.

The middle six chapters delineate the essential message of the Bhagavad-gita: *bhakti-yoga*, or connection with the Supreme through pure love. In essence, spirituality is a matter of the heart, but that doesn't mean we don't employ the head. In Chapter Seven, entitled 'Knowledge of the Absolute,' Krishna establishes the need to attentively hear the messages of the Supreme Person. Through this process of hearing, one can awaken expansive, untainted, divine knowledge, otherwise inaccessible to limited human perception. This knowledge acts as a lamp in the dark enclosure of the material world – it guides one to the exit door, and simultaneously reveals everything that will be encountered on the route there. Through descending knowledge we ascend beyond the mistakes we are otherwise inevitably prone to.

In the holy land of Vrindavana, Lord Krishna, in His divine play as a cowherd boy, daily takes the cows and calves out to graze. To gather them at the end of the day He employs different techniques. First He lovingly calls their names. For those that don't hear, He plays His enchanting flute. Some cows remain estranged, and His next step it to loudly blow His buffalo horn. If, despite all these efforts, the cows and calves still don't return, He goes out with a stick to chase them back!

Just like the cows, we have strayed from our spiritual home-base. First class intelligence can grasp the truth simply by hearing divine knowledge, assimilating the teachings and arriving at the mature conclusion without need for anything more. Second class intelligence requires a visual demonstration – the need to observe a real-life example which illustrates the teachings. Third class intelligence is activated only by directly experiencing the teachings through events and interactions in our own life. Failure to learn through these avenues causes a return to the School of Hard Knocks, the material world, where the soul commences a new chapter of life. Unless spirituality is awakened, their activities, and the subsequent mistakes they make, perpetually entangle them in an expansive network of *karma*. Thus, to avoid mistakes, we have to access and embrace the eternal truths that come from conscientious hearing.

"Out of many thousands among men, one may endeavour for perfection, and of those who have achieved perfection, hardly one knows Me in truth."

(Bhagavad-gita 7.3)

References

7.1 – The science of hearing spiritual knowledge.

Learning through Hearing

Can you think of something you were taught by hearing, but only really learnt deeply after experiencing?

Can you think of something that you learnt by hearing that saved you from having to personally experience it?

Why do you think we don't learn from hearing? List all the reasons and then identify which ones particularly relate to yourself.

Is there anything you have heard recently that you could learn from and apply in your life?

how to face death

8

Srila Prabhupada was once asked why the death rate in India was so high. His reply - *"The death rate is the same everywhere I go - 100%!"* A witty but sobering response. Time and tide wait for no man, and indeed, no man makes it out alive. Throughout the Vedic literatures we find detailed accounts of how great personalities left this world. The final lesson of their life reminds us of how to face the inevitability of death with grace, detachment and spiritual consciousness. While leaving this world, these great personalities leave behind profound teachings and an inspiring example to follow.

In Chapter Eight of the Bhagavad-gita, Krishna explains how a person's thoughts at the time of death sum up their consciousness and aspirations cultivated throughout life. Thus, one's state of mind at the critical moment of departure determines the next life situation - those who remember God at death reach the kingdom of God. One may spend decades at school, but if they're lazy, inattentive and apathetic in their studies, they won't pass the final exam. They'll have to retake. Similarly, the success of life is measured by how well we perform in the final exam; death. How we perform in the final exam is largely dependent on how diligently we prepare ourselves during the course of life. We must live with the end in mind.

The thought of death, though shocking for many, need not be seen as an inconvenient truth, but rather the ultimate meditation to reinstate clarity and perspective into every aspect of our life. Consider the following:

Priority - death reminds us of our priorities; those critical things we have to pursue before time runs out. Knowing we have to leave behind our possessions, positions and profiles, pushes us to invest in our spiritual wealth which remains our eternal asset.

Urgency - death not only reminds us of what is important, but urges us to pursue it now. We're impelled to overcome procrastination - there's no point in killing time once you realise that time is actually killing you.

Humility – death fosters a deep sense of humility. Our utter powerlessness in counteracting death helps us realise we're not in control and higher powers are at work. The annihilation of pride opens doors to heightened spiritual realisation.

Clarity - through the lens of temporality, we perceive everything and everyone we complain about in a new light. We all have the experience of failing to appreciate things until they have gone. In presence we tend to focus on negatives, but in absence we see significant value.

Immunity - in the face of permanent expiry, all of our worries and anxieties pale into insignificance. Life is full of many fears, but our greatest fear is of death, before which all others pale in comparison. Being fearless of death immunises us from fear altogether.

Opportunity – death is a portal to new opportunities, a gateway to our true existence and nature. It's not something negative or destructive; it is the opposite - hugely life affirming.

"After attaining Me, the great souls, who are yogis in devotion, never return to this temporary world, which is full of miseries, because they have attained the highest perfection."

(Bhagavad-gita 8.15)

References

8.27 – Those engaged in spiritual life become fearless of death.

Life's Change Agent

Imagine you receive a message from a close friend that they only have one month left to live. Based on what you have learnt about 'How to Face Death,' write an encouraging and empowering letter to them which:

- Helps them understand the spiritual perspective behind death
- Addresses their fears, anxieties and insecurities
- Offers ideas and advice on how to utilise their remaining time
- Gives an uplifting sense of hope, positivity, inspiration

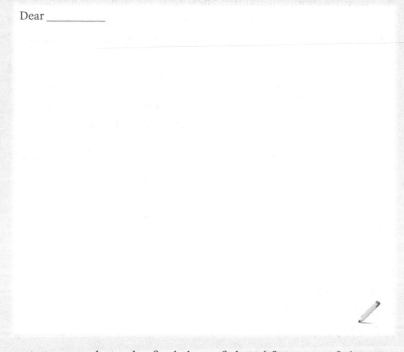

Dear _____

Assisting people in the final days of their life is one of the most powerful contributions you can make. When those who are facing this predicament are assisted by individuals who have spiritual depth, emotional maturity and practical sensitivity, the most difficult time of their life can become the most rewarding.

9 how to find **Love**

Industries thrive on it, popstars sing about it, teenagers dream about it, and people are willing to do just about anything for it. To love and be loved – the everlasting, universal dream. Unfortunately, though we wholeheartedly endeavour for that perfect connection in our material sojourn, for the most part it's a let-down, and the story of life is more a case of *frustrated* love.

But do we truly know what love even is? We freely say *"I love you,"* but if we don't deeply understand our own identity, the identity of the person we profess such feelings for, and how love is actually defined, how seriously can we take the statement? Thus, ancient literatures begin by clarifying who we really are – spiritual beings in temporary bodies. This helps us understand that true love goes beyond the physical and emotional, and is rather based on spiritual connection. Furthermore, the literatures delineate what love is – an outpouring of heartfelt service which is entirely unmotivated (*ahaituki*) and uninterrupted (*apratihata*). Such loving exchange brings fulfilment to the soul (*yenatma suprasidati*).

Chapter Nine falls right in the middle of the sacred dialogue, and Krishna reserves this prime spot for the most confidential knowledge. When we selflessly give ourselves in a relationship, the strength of that loving sentiment conquers the heart of the other. This power of purity is so irresistible that it even captures the attention of the Supreme Lord. Krishna declares that even the most simple things in existence, a leaf, fruit, flower or water, if offered with genuine and sincere love, conquer His heart.

When the innate desire for loving connection is reposed in Krishna, not only is that love perfectly reciprocated with, but it's also abundantly distributed. Our 'loving' connections in this world are often the cause of the greatest pain due to feelings of let-down and lack of reciprocation. When those powerful emotions are directed toward Krishna without any ulterior motive we experience the most perfect loving reciprocation. As Srila Prabhupada says: *"If we make our friendship with Krishna, it will never break. If we make our master Krishna, we will never be cheated. If we love Krishna as our son, He will never die. If we love Krishna as our lover, He will be the best of all, and there will be no separation. Because Krishna is the Supreme Lord, He is unlimited and has an unlimited number of devotees."*

Furthermore, since Krishna is the source of all, the love we offer to Him naturally flows towards everyone and everything. As a light directed into a diamond is reflected in all directions, when we have love for Krishna, all our other relationships become infused by the devotional connection and we become empowered to exponentially widen our circle of love. Thus, by loving Krishna, we let our love break free from its limitations and flow unimpeded, bringing supreme happiness in our own lives and the lives of many others.

By learning to love in this realm, we prepare ourselves to enter the ultimate realm of pure love: *"Real love is in the spiritual world between Radha and Krishna. Real love is between Krishna and the gopis. Real love, the friendship is there between Krishna and His cowherd boys. Real love between animal and man is there–Krishna is loving the cows and calves. Real love between trees, flowers, water. Simply that is the platform of love. That is spiritual world. Everything love."* (Srila Prabhupada)

"I envy no one, nor am I partial to anyone. I am equal to all. But whoever renders service unto Me in devotion is a friend, is in Me, and I am also a friend to him."

(Bhagavad-gita 9.29)

References

9.29 – When one approaches Krishna, He reciprocates in a very personal way.

Loving Connections

Think of an important relationship in your life. Ask yourself the following questions:

How do you see that individual and what is the basis of your relationship with them?

What behaviours / attitudes block that relationship from blossoming, and what could you do to change that?

How could you incorporate more spirituality into the relationship so it's based on a higher principle?

What would selfless service look like in this relationship?

how to perceive beauty

10

Whether a beautiful person, place or piece of artwork, they all have a magnetic pull that captures our imagination. Knowing this, we invest so much in trying to own that beauty so we can attract and enchant others! Last year, US consumers spent $154 million dollars on nail polish, $278 million on eye makeup, $291 million on lipstick, and $12.4 billion on plastic surgery. The trend continues, with no sign of easing.

In Chapter Ten, Krishna explains that behind all the beauty of the world stands the all-attractive and enchanting Personality of Godhead. The word *bhagavan*, indicating God, literally means He whose qualities are so charming that everyone is irresistibly drawn to invest themselves in Him. Why then, one may wonder, are we drawn to the beauty of this world? Because, Krishna says, everything beautiful in this world springs from but a spark of His splendour! We can look at an attractive person and consider: *"If they are that beautiful, imagine how beautiful the creator is!"*

Some see the material world as an object of enjoyment – they look **AT** the world. This is known as the path of *karma*. Because they approach the various aspects of material nature with a view of exploitation, everything backfires. For those who embody this selfish, enjoying spirit, Krishna rubber stamps the material world as temporary and miserable (*dukhalayam asasvatam*). When we look AT the world, we are looking for the right thing (happiness), but in the wrong place, and in the wrong way.

Others see the material world as an illusion – they look **AWAY** from the world. In a world where leaders are brainless, politics is shameless, people are heartless and desires are endless, they conclude that everything is useless! Having been frustrated in their attempts to enjoy the world, they become averse and desire to escape the world. This can lead to an impersonal vision where they label the entire creation as an illusion, and instead aspire to enter an eternal nothingness. The Bhagavad-gita, however, clarifies that though the material world is temporary and unsubstantial, it is not unreal. A photocopy may lack the clarity, quality and colour of the original, but it's still a real document that provides information. In the same way, the material world, though lacking the fullness of the spiritual world, has its part to play and can render us great benefit if we interact with it appropriately.

The *bhakti-yogis* look **BEYOND** the world. They see it as a bridge leading to our true home, and things within it can be appropriately engaged for the purpose of pleasing Krishna. Devotees find a way to interact with the world which elevates themselves and others. This is known as *yukta-vairagya*, or the process of engaging worldly things for a higher cause and spiritual purpose. The *bhakti-yogis* see the world, but on the backdrop of eternity.

It would be crazy to say there is no beauty in this world. That beauty keeps the world revolving, as people run around madly in pursuance of it. Rather than avoiding it, spiritualists learn to acknowledge it, appreciate it and contextualise it. Instead of trying to exploit or ignore that beauty, they engage that beauty in the service of the most beautiful, and in that way get connected to the source of all beauty.

"Know that all opulent, beautiful and glorious creations spring from but a spark of My splendour."

(Bhagavad-gita 10.41)

References

10.41 – All beauty comes from Krishna.

Enjoy, Ignore or Engage?

Think of a beautiful person, place and object. For each one describe the approach, behaviour and attitude of someone who tries to enjoy, ignore or engage appropriately:

	Person	Place	Object
Description			
Try to Enjoy it			
Try to Ignore it			
Try to engage it			

Question: As spiritualists is there scope to sometimes enjoy things, and sometimes opt to ignore things? What are the dangers in trying to engage worldly things for spiritual growth, and in what situations might that end up being detrimental?

■how to■ detect ■
divinity

11

The world we live in today has drawn an aggressive demarcation between science and spirituality. According to this fabricated dichotomy, anyone who is scientific can only really operate in the realms of physicalism, and anyone who is spiritual can never really be objective and scientific in their approach. This notion, however, needs critical reassessment.

The *bhakti* teachers have meticulously established that spiritual processes to uncover higher states of consciousness are systematic, replicable, measurable and practical. Not only that, but there are clear and observable signs and symptoms which indicate the efficacy of one's practice and act as reference points for the spiritual scientist. These practices and symptoms are not just internal and subtle, but externally visible and tangible. Interestingly, Srila Prabhupada's masterful summary study of Bhakti-Rasamrta-Sindhu, a handbook on devotion, is subtitled 'The Complete Science of Devotion.'

Though *bhakti-yoga* is scientific, it is not mechanical. The elements of grace, consciousness, subjective expression and personal individuality cannot be eliminated from the equation. *Bhakti* practitioners are not passionate *achievers* but rather humble and grateful *receivers*. This doesn't jeopardise the scientific status of *bhakti*, but encourages us to broaden our definition. We need to appreciate that it is indeed a *higher-dimensional* science.

In Chapter Eleven, Krishna manifests a divine display before Arjuna by showing His Universal Form. While Krishna could be externally mistaken as your average Jo, when He exhibits the Universal Form, His Divinity and Supremacy become crystal clear. Arjuna is flabbergasted and he requests Krishna to again assume His humanlike form, which is far more lovable and relatable. God is great, but God is also sweet, and it's this intimacy of relationship that we seek more than anything.

The incidents of this chapter serve to remind the reader that not just anyone can claim to be God. When the Lord descends He is predicted in scripture, identified by astrological calculation, verified by the great teachers, and ultimately, displays extraordinary, super-human acts. This gives us a frame work within which to scrutinise any claims of divinity that may surface. Beyond this, however, the Supreme Person reveals Himself in response to our own heartfelt practice and engagement in spiritual science.

Bhakti is a science which is not experimental but rather experiential – a higher grade science which fine tunes the consciousness so one is able to detect divinity and experience tangible reciprocation with God. Great teachers have documented a sensible process of devotional practice that culminates in divine love. Scientific, calculated spiritual practices (in Sanskrit, *sadhana-bhakti*) performed with enthusiasm, patience and determination, usher one towards the spiritual reality. Eventually, we are able to relate to God, just as we would relate to anyone around us. That's the real proof that we're all looking for.

"If You think that I am able to behold Your cosmic form, O my Lord, O master of all mystic power, then kindly show me that unlimited universal Self."

(Bhagavad-gita 11.4)

References

11.54 – Only by undivided devotion can one actually find God.

11.55 – How one can transform all activities so they support one's divine connection.

Connection Points

In the ancient treatise of devotion written by Rupa Goswami, known as Bhakti-Rasamrita-Sindhu, he outlines 64 ways in which one's devotional connection with Krishna can be reawakened. Amongst them he stresses five to be the most powerful:

Spiritual People (*sadhu-sanga*) – association with spiritually minded people.

Spiritual Books (*bhagavata-sravana*) – study and immersion in spiritual literature.

Spiritual Sounds (*nama-kirtan*) – meditation and absorption in the divine name of Krishna.

Spiritual Places (*mathura-vasa*) – visits to and residence in places of pilgrimage.

Spiritual Forms (*murti-seva*) – practical service to the personal deity form of God.

What can you do to engage in these five spiritually powerful acts on a regular basis.

	Once a week	Once a month	Once a year
Spiritual People			
Spiritual Books			
Spiritual Sounds			
Spiritual Places			
Spiritual Objects			

how to spiritually
pr●gress

If you want to take someone somewhere, first you have to meet them where they are. It's a simple but often overlooked point. This principle stands universal – in education, in parenting, in leadership, in marketing, and even in the development of spirituality. One reason why the Vedic tradition is considered the most advanced theology in existence is because of its multi-level ingenuity. Though it clearly establishes the ultimate goal, the apex of spiritual consciousness, it simultaneously offers multiple options of spiritual practice for those unable to immediately grasp the most elevated level of purity. Although the goal is one, the steps of progress toward it are numerous.

In Chapter Twelve, which constitutes the final of the *Bhakti* chapters, Krishna gives a flavour of His magnanimity and flexibility. Having established unalloyed devotion (*bhakti-yoga*) as the most evolved path of spirituality, He goes on to offer other options, recognising that this heartfelt connection may not be within everyone's immediate grasp. Progressive steps towards such a pure devotional spirit include the practice of regulated spirituality, worship through one's daily work, offering of charity, and the cultivation of knowledge. The spiritual path is not all or nothing and one can begin their journey according to what is appealing and achievable.

Elsewhere in the Gita, Krishna talks about worship of demigods, impersonalism and the even the practice of pantheism. When we look at the world we see that the majority of people may not be searching for pure, unalloyed love, but rather have many other 'not-so-spiritual' desires in mind. Thus, different types of worship allow one to fulfill their material aspirations and simultaneously step onto the 'spiritual ladder.' For example, worship of various 'demigods' to attain wealth, health and prosperity is sometimes prescribed. Such worship and practice, over a period of time, will bring the practitioner to a more refined and elevated sense of spirituality, where they completely divorce themselves from worldly pursuits. In maturity, they arrive at the point of desiring an unmotivated relationship and reciprocation with the one Supreme God.

The best teachers deeply understand the needs, interests and concerns of the audience they teach. They expertly address those aspirations in a way that simultaneously elevates their spiritual status. One size never fits all, and teaching has to be tailor-made and personalised. This gives great hope to students who may see the ultimate goal as way beyond their reach. The teachers will remind them about what perfection looks like, but consistently focus on progression forward from the point they are currently at.

This insight is invaluable for our own spiritual journey. Often there is a gap between the ideal and the real – where we are, and what the ultimate goal actually is. These gaps can sometimes feel uncomfortable. The practical and incremental steps forward that Krishna offers bolster our hope and optimism that reaching the ideal is not a utopian aspiration. We have to start where we are, use what we have and do what we can. Progress brings perfection.

"My dear Arjuna, O winner of wealth, if you cannot fix your mind upon Me without deviation, then follow the regulative principles of bhakti-yoga. In this way develop a desire to attain Me."

(Bhagavad-gita 12.9)

References

12.8-12 – Multiple stages and options that Krishna offers for spiritual progression.

Spiritual Flow

The art of growth is to bend ourselves without breaking ourselves. The tendency in life is to underachieve or overstretch. When the challenge level exceeds our capacity level we end up breaking down. When our capacity level exceeds the challenge level, we stagnate in the comfort zone. Thus, we have to keep progressing by building our capacity, and simultaneously finding appropriate goals and challenges to meet that skill level.

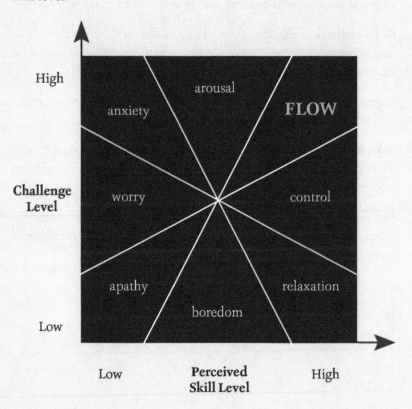

In order to find that flow state, here are some general tips:

Set Goals – this give you a sense of achievement and also allows you to gauge your present capacity, and how that is growing over time

Get Feedback – ask experienced spiritual practitioners for advice and share with them your goals for growth so they can add their experiences into the equation

Invest in Yourself – increase your capacity by learning and evolving, so that you can take on bigger challenges

Take Risks – don't be afraid to take risks and try something different – whether it 'works' or not, it will certainly give you more insight and understanding about yourself and your potential

Be Steady – in order to build spiritual momentum and have cumulative effect, and the principle is never to take a step down. Growth should be pursued in such a way that it never takes you back.

13 how to find freedom

Let me tell you the story of Stanislavsky Lech. The Nazis stormed into his home one night and herded him and his family into a death camp in Krakow. His loved ones were murdered, one by one, day by day, before his eyes. Weak, grieving, and starving, he worked from sunrise to sundown alongside the other prisoners of the concentration camp, destined for the same. How could anyone survive such horrors? Somehow he continued.

One day, he looked at the nightmare around him and understood that if he continued in this fashion, he would die. He resolved that he had to escape. Although no one before him had ever escaped, he fostered the belief that somehow there was a way. His focus changed from how to survive, to instead asking, *"How can we escape from this terrible place?"* His fellow inmates offered no encouragement. *"Don't be a fool! There is no escape. Asking such questions will only torture your soul."* Lech wouldn't accept this answer. His constant meditation was, *"How can I do it? There must be a way. How can I get out of here?"*

One day, Lech smelled rotting flesh just a few feet from where he worked. He peered over a large boundary wall and saw a horrific sight: men, women, and children who had been gassed and whose naked corpses lay there in a human mountain. Instead of focusing on the question *"How could God allow something so evil to happen?"* he asked himself, *"How can I use this to escape?"* As the sun set and the work party left for the barracks, he pulled off his clothes and dove naked into the pile of bodies while no one was looking. Pretending to be dead, he waited with the sickening smell of death all around him, the weight of all the corpses pressing upon him. Finally, he heard a truck engine start. After a short ride, the mountain of bodies was dumped into an open grave. He waited until all vehicles had departed, and then ran - naked - twenty five miles to freedom.

What made the difference between the fate of Stanislavsky Lech and that of everyone else who died in concentration camps? Likely several factors, but one key lesson was that he asked a *different* question. That curiosity became his meditation, a reference point for everything he observed. He asked it repeatedly, certain he would receive an answer. Our questions influence our focus, how we think and feel, and what we see. Asking powerful questions can be a major way to turn our life around. Instead of asking, *"Why is life so unfair?"* and *"How can I eclipse that person?"* we could reengineer our questions in order to elicit answers that will really help us progress.

In Chapter Thirteen, Arjuna asks Krishna to define six subjects: *prakrti* (nature), *purusa* (the enjoyer), *ksetra* (the field of activities), *ksetrajna* (the knower of the field), *jnanam* (knowledge and the process of knowing), and *jneyam* (the object of knowledge). These subjects are key elements of Vedic philosophy and Krishna therefore spends the entire chapter defining and discussing them. Arjuna, although an established transcendentalist, plays the part of a materially entangled individual so he can pose questions for the benefit of humanity. His astute inquiries create the opportunity for Krishna to offer answers to life's most profound mysteries. Perfect questions and perfect answers – a dialogue that opens the doors to freedom on the highest plane. Now ask yourself, what questions am I asking in life?

"One who understands this philosophy concerning material nature, the living entity and the interaction of the modes of nature is sure to attain liberation. He will not take birth here again, regardless of his present position."

(Bhagavad-gita 13.24)

References

13.1-2 – Arjuna's inquiries and why these aspects of reality are so crucial to understand.

Big Questions

Respond to the following questions and search deeply for the most authentic answer that comes to mind:

1. If you woke up tomorrow with no fear what would you do first?

2. Of the things you take for granted every day, what is most valuable?

3. Think of the happiest and most content time in your life, and now question why that was?

4. If you could make a ten second speech to the entire world, what would you say?

5. What would you do differently if you knew nobody would judge you?

6. In your life, what are you holding onto that you need to let go of?

7. Do I care more about how my life looks or how it feels?

8. If you had to teach something what would you teach?

Look closely at your answers. For many questions you may have struggled to find an answer. Look at the answers you have come up with and question how much they resonate with what is deep within you.

At another time, perhaps in a peaceful and secluded surrounding, take an hour and ask yourself these questions again. Unpack them and brainstorm, and you will find you gain more clarity about what sits deep within you.

14 how to avoid burnout

Burnout is more common than ever; physical and mental levels of activity become unsustainable and we're forced to retire out of exhaustion. Not only does it dent our ability to meet our goals and realise our dreams, but the perceived failure creates an inner feeling of defeat and dejection and can permanently damage our morale. The ancient scriptures give three broad principles for avoiding burnout, and, on the positive side, discovering a space where you can thrive:

Do the Right *Things* – Follow your *dharma*

Adopt the Right *Lifestyle* – Live in *sattva*

Embody the Right *Motivation* – Act with *prema*

Our *dharma*, as previously discussed, refers to our unique psychophysical nature. When we work and function outside of our *dharma* we fail to utilise our strengths and compensate for our weaknesses, and thus become susceptible to burnout. *Prema* denotes 'love' - we should aspire for a life where that love drives what we do. We should work for a cause that genuinely moves our heart. It's crucial to resonate with and have feeling for what we do, and not just work for immediate benefits like money, position, accolade and security.

Now let's explore *sattva*. In Chapter Fourteen, Krishna expands upon the concept of the three modes, explaining how a lifestyle built on *sattva* is beneficial from all angles of vision. What we see on a TV screen is an intricate interaction of pixels in three basic colours - red, blue and yellow. They combine in endless combinations to produce images and scenes which enchant our minds. In the same way, the material world, and everything within it, is essentially composed of the three modes of nature - goodness (*sattva*), passion (*rajas*) and ignorance (*tamas*). Everything surrounding us is made of different permutations of these modes, and that in turn creates a permutation within us.

This framework is powerful, practical and so universal that, when comprehensively understood, can be applied to virtually any aspect of life. How one parents their children, the food we eat, the environment we create around us, the style of leadership and management we adopt, the way we drive our car – everything can, and should, be done in *sattva* for maximum wellbeing.

When we live in *sattva* we maximise our achievements. The food we eat gives copious amounts of energy and vitality, our leadership brings the best out of the people we serve, and our driving is safe, cost-effective and efficient. Furthermore, on an internal level, living in *sattva* creates an inner harmony and groove that allows us to sustain our activity without becoming fatigued, imbalanced or overwhelmed. When we live in *sattva*, we guard ourselves against the potential of burnout, which is a natural characteristic of the mode of passion.

"From the mode of goodness, real knowledge develops; from the mode of passion, greed develops; and from the mode of ignorance develop foolishness, madness and illusion."

(Bhagavad-gita 14.17)

References

14.5-9 – Fundamental definitions of the three modes of material nature.

14.10 – How the modes are constantly fluctuating and competing.

Sattva Life

The three modes are like the three primary colours - yellow, red, and blue. Just as one can mix red, yellow, and blue at different proportions to produce millions of colours, the modes of nature mix with each other to create the variety we see in the world.

The Gita discusses how the modes influence a person's character, behaviour, and approach to life. Goodness leads to lasting happiness – it often begins by tasting like poison, requiring one to sacrifice and regulate, but ends up tasting like nectar. Passion brings short-term happiness that begins like nectar but ends like poison. The mode of ignorance (at best) leads to happiness that is illusory in both the long and the short term, being the result of laziness, idleness, and negligence.

With reference to the Gita's teachings, what would someone's approach to the following things look like based on the predominant mode they are operating in:

	Goodness (*sattva*)	Passion (*rajas*)	Ignorance (*tamas*)
Food	Gives strength, health, happiness and satisfaction	Too bitter, pungent, hot, dry – causes disease	Tasteless, decomposed and putrid
Time of day	12.00am-8.00am	8.00am-4.00pm	4.00pm-12.00am
Sleeping			
Parenting			
Driving			
Discussion			
House Environment			
Spiritual Practices			

(15) how to become detached

Srila Prabhupada once boldly stated that the guru knows *everything*. The reporter then asked him how many windows the Empire State Building had. Srila Prabhupada gravely looked back and countered, *"How many drops of water in a mirage?"* What a brilliant answer! Amidst constant change, can we identify anything in this world to be really real? Although not illusory, this realm is most definitely temporary. For this reason, Vedic scriptures describe this physical world as unreal. Although it can be perceived by our human senses, it is constantly changing and has no endurance in the context of eternity.

In the final chapters of the Bhagavad-gita, one of Krishna's prime objectives is to engender a sense of detachment within Arjuna and the reader. In Chapter Fifteen, He compares the material world to the reflection of a banyan tree in water. In Sanskrit, the banyan tree is known as *asvattha* which etymologically means *'That which will not be here tomorrow.'* Though discussing the temporality of the world and everything within it may sound depressing, it's actually incredibly empowering. By awakening this sense of detachment we recalibrate our vision and begin to focus on the enduring spiritual reality.

As spiritual beings we're not residents of London, Lagos or Los Angeles, but rather residents of the spiritual world. One must undoubtedly attend to the immediate demands, pressures and responsibilities of life, lest we become dysfunctional members of society. One would do well, however, to avoid becoming overly engrossed and captivated by the temporal affairs of daily life. As a wise spiritualist once quipped *"Don't take the illusion too seriously!"*

The world teaches us to base our sense of identity and self-worth on transitory, external and artificial considerations. When we identify with our abilities, facilities and positions of responsibility, then we set ourselves up for crisis. Why? Because the indisputable nature of this world is that such things will almost always fade away over time.

We pride ourselves in our 'unique' abilities but eventually our faculties decline, we witness our own ineptitude, or we find someone far more qualified and competent who supersedes us. Painful! We treasure our karmic gifts like beauty, physique, learning and wealth – but the waves of time callously carry them away. Painful! We feel valuable because of our reputation, influence and position in society – but everyone has 'their day,' after which we all have to make way. Painful! Constant change is the underlying theme of the material phantasmagoria – it's unstoppable, unpredictable and uncontrollable. Thus, we suffer a subtle ego death every time we falsely identify with the temporary.

Thus, wisdom teachers continually remind us to focus on our eternal and unchanging identity. As spiritual beings, our true ego lies in being a selfless servant of God. Everything we receive in the journey of life is simply a facility and detail in pursuance of this, with any given situation always offering a unique opportunity for selfless service. In such detached spiritual consciousness, all anxiety, fear and dissatisfaction disappears.

"The real form of this tree cannot be perceived in this world. No one can understand where it ends, where it begins, or where its foundation is. But with determination one must cut down this strongly rooted tree with the weapon of detachment."

(Bhagavad-gita 15.3)

References

15.3-4 – Becoming detached from the material world.

Eternal Assets

In material consciousness, we feel self-worth and a sense of identity based on:

Abilities – things we do which give us a sense of achievement

Facilities – things that help us function and fulfil our desires

Positions – roles and relationships that give a sense of control and contribution

Have you experienced how the above things can be taken away, sometimes in quite unpredictable ways? How did that, or would that, make you feel? Can you think of abilities, facilities and positions that you can identify with which are more spiritual in nature and can never be taken away from you? How would life be if you built your identity on those spiritual, unchanging, things?

	What do you identify with?	How has / could this be taken away?	What could be a spiritual version of this that you could more identify with?
Abilities			
Facilities			
Positions			

how to
change
outlook

16

High streets are intriguing places: a microcosm of modern life. It's where people descend in their thousands, searching for something special to enrich their existence. These urban hubs are a melting pot of entertainers, campaigners, shoppers, beggars and advertisers, a marketplace for the latest commodities and ideas, a space for meeting, sharing and exploring. As a monk I spent many years travelling up and down the country, standing in town centres, speaking to random people and showing them spiritual books. It's quite a task to stop someone in their tracks, cut through the myriad of thoughts, penetrate the bubble of their life and begin a dialogue about deeper subject matter. But truly amazing - some of my most mystical, memorable and moving experiences in life have been in bustling high streets, sharing spirituality with everyday people.

On one particular day, in minus degree temperatures, a homeless beggar sat on the sidewalk holding a ragged sign which read *'Give me hope.'* Over the years I had become desensitised to it, although it was a harsh reality way beyond my world of comprehension. Seeing him sleeping rough, a few people threw in some coins, someone else gifted him a Costa coffee, while an occasional passer-by stopped to offer a few comforting words. All nice gestures. But, my heart said, what he really needs is *hope*. In that sense we are all beggars – we all need hope. Without the conviction of a brighter future what drives us to continue on in this world? Hope, faith, inspiration and vision, which give us the hunger for life, are perhaps our most precious assets – if we have those, we have everything. In that spirit I gifted him a bag of food and a spiritual book, serving the immediate but trying to address the ultimate, hoping it would uplift his outlook.

In Chapter Sixteen, Krishna explains the divine and demoniac natures, their mentalities, activities and destinies. Everything, however, stems from their philosophy – their outlook on life. Some individuals see through the eyes of divine wisdom, and that sets them on a certain trajectory. Others, however, see through tainted material vision – blurred, blinded and short-sighted. Connecting with spiritual wisdom is something that changes our outlook entirely, endowing one with the x-ray vision to see beyond the superficial.

Modern psychology tells us our outlook on life is moulded by two broad factors. Our 'nature' is the inbred specific mentality and psychophysical conditions we carry with us from previous lives. Everyone is wired differently because of the journey they've been on, each with our own strengths and weaknesses. In addition to this is 'nurture' - our interaction in this life. The people, places, opinions and situations we encounter throughout life, shape our outlook.

The sages explain, however, that there is a third dimension which can create a paradigm shift in our approach to life. Our *condition* from previous lives (nature) and *interaction* in this life (nurture) may well set the stage, but our *connection* with spiritual wisdom can be the game-changer. It helps us to step back and observe our inbred nature and lifetime of nurture. It loosens our identification with the temporary, and can awaken the innate pure consciousness which can shine beyond the subtle, material impressions we all carry. That transcendent dimension brings a deeper purpose, divine presence and irresistible empowerment that shifts our consciousness entirely.

"He who discards scriptural injunctions and acts according to his own whims attains neither perfection, nor happiness, nor the supreme destination."

(Bhagavad-gita 16.23)

References

16.9 – The outlook of those who deny God's existence.

16.10 – How that outlook can have destructive effects on the world.

True Lies

Nature and Nurture can cement us in a worldview and way of thinking that's not necessarily in line with reality. We carry many biases within us, which can limit and impede our growth and progress. Consider the following and reflect on whether you can pinpoint examples of them in your life? Can you then think of examples where connection with spiritual wisdom has helped you to overcome or see beyond those biases?

Five Popular Biases

Framing Bias – the tendency to accept information or opinions that are presented in a language and style with which we resonate.

Anchoring Bias – the tendency to be overly influenced by the first piece of information that we receive.

Consensus Bias – the tendency to accept the opinions and understanding of the people that immediately surround us.

Attentional Bias – the tendency for recurring thoughts to skew one's perception and cement one into a way of thinking.

Self-Serving Bias – the tendency to believe those things which serve our personal desires, needs and motivations.

	An example of this in your life?	How was this bias exposed?
Framing Bias		
Anchoring Bias		
Consensus Bias		
Attentional Bias		
Self-Serving Bias		

how to perfect your
speech

17

Our modern world suffers from over-communication. The prevailing culture insists we reply to all text messages within 10 minutes, be attentive to the mountain of emails building up in our inbox, and religiously return random 'missed calls' on our phones. Don't forget to regularly post something witty on Instagram, follow obscure acquaintances on Twitter, and utilise all the free airtime minutes on your mobile contract! It is, after all, good to talk. *But what is the net result of this web of exchange? Does it foster a greater sense of relationship and community, or is it a case of electronically connected, but further apart?*

Silence, it's said, is the art of conversation. You may have noticed how we struggle with a quiet moment. When it does arise, most will instinctively grab their smartphone in a desperate attempt to occupy their mind. Think about the last time you saw a young adult sitting down and doing absolutely nothing. Rare indeed! Even more unusual is to be with another person and not utter a word. It feels awkward and uneasy; alien and unnerving. Yet silence is essential – it forces us to understand, assimilate, reflect and think deeply about what is actually going on. Often times, however, in order to frantically fill those vacant moments, we end up generating substandard content to share with the world: meaningless, inconsiderate and shoddy communication.

Of all skills, the ability to appropriately utilise our speech is amongst the most powerful. In Chapter Seventeen, Krishna offers an over-arching model to guide our discourse. Words, He recommends, should be truthful, pleasing and beneficial. According to ancient legend, Socrates was once approached by someone bursting to express something. Before he could utter a word, Socrates questioned whether what he was itching to say was definitely true. The man was unsure. *"No matter,"* Socrates said *"Is it something pleasant?"* The man told him it wasn't – likely a controversy or scandal. Socrates asked him one last question – *"Is what you're about to tell me something which will benefit and improve the situation?"* The man now realised what Socrates was teaching him. If what we speak is neither true, nor pleasing, nor beneficial, it's best it remains unsaid. In Plato's words, *"Wise men speak because they have something to say; fools because they have to say something!"*

How much of our written and verbal communication would make it through this filter? Don't get me wrong, there is definitely room for chitchat, niceties, and light-hearted exchange between humans. It would be unnatural to jump to the extreme of strictly regulating our every word. Along with freedom of speech, however, it may be worthwhile to remind people of their longstanding right to freedom of thought. Our words should educate, encourage and empower others, leaving a positive feeling and tangible sense of upliftment.

I always remember a mentor and friend who would tell me – *"If all the words you said today were written over your body, would you still look like a saintly person?"* A powerful meditation to embed within our psyche to help us filter out the nonsense.

"Austerity of speech consists in speaking words that are truthful, pleasing, beneficial, and not agitating to others, and also in regularly reciting Vedic literature."

(Bhagavad-gita 17.15)

References

17.15 – The principles of powerful speech.

Real Conversations

The Bhagavad-gita is not just a theological classic but a practical guidebook. The dialogue actually reveals the principles of powerful conversation, an art that's fast disappearing. Look around and observe people talking – often, they are disconnected, disinterested and disengaged, and even when they manage to draw each other in, nothing valuable or productive is really generated from all the natter. Knowing how to have a good conversation is an indispensable life skill.

Consider the following points and draw from experiences where you have followed or neglected these principles:

Attention – Despite the fever-pitch intensity of the battlefield, Arjuna managed to shut everything out and give his undivided attention to Krishna. Attention, they say, is the rarest and purest form of generosity. It pays to be fully present in any dialogue, since your counterpart will wholeheartedly work overtime to reciprocate with your investment.

Openness – Arjuna was open to suggestion. *"I am a student,"* he said, *"please offer feedback and guide me."* That's progressive. If you enter a conversation fixated on what you'll say and what you want to hear, you paralyse the process of discovery. Let the person express their heart, and be ready to wholeheartedly receive. Temporarily suspend your personal opinion and let your perspective be challenged.

Spontaneity – Arjuna was baffled and bewildered, looking for answers but lacking clarity and structure. Krishna patiently responded to his every inquiry, taking the hour-long conversation through twists and turns, and full circle! Good conversations go with the flow. Often times it's more valuable to ditch the planned route in your head, and instead talk about what is lingering deep within. Then we get to the heart of the issue.

Honesty – Arjuna lays all the cards on the table. He has doubts, questions, disagreements and issues, and he eventually reveals it all. In response to his honesty, Krishna offers gem-like insights. When you are real with people, they'll be real with you, and then it gets 'real interesting.' Superficiality is the breeding ground of the most uninteresting interactions.

Humility – Hearing Arjuna's request for guidance, Krishna is reluctant. Even after Krishna offers His flawless advice, He states this is merely *"His opinion"* and encourages Arjuna to *"do as he wishes to do."* Krishna's humility is revealing. Conversations are not a platform for self-promotion or proving ourselves; it's not about winning or defeating. In a conversation, don't simply listen so you can reply, but listen to genuinely understand.

18

how to
conquer

fear

Fear can easily overshadow our life. Of course, there is an instinctive fear which is absolutely necessary for survival - it's good to be scared if a car is heading straight for you at 100mph! Aside from this, however, are the artificial fears that plague us from morning to evening, irrational thoughts taken out of perspective which hijack our consciousness. *Can you think of a fear you have now that you didn't have twenty years ago? Can you think of a fear from your youth that you've managed to overcome? Can you think of a fear you have that someone else is oblivious to?* The affirmative answer in each case proves something extremely powerful - fear is something which is learnt, and that means it can also be unlearnt. Fear is an imposition.

We have fears about the world, fears about our health, fears about our family and friends, fears about the future and fears of failure. When we're happy we're fearful it may end. When we're sad we're fearful it may never end! I once saw a bumper sticker which read, *'Do not disturb... already disturbed!'* In Chapter One, Arjuna was certainly grappling with fear. Faced with the prospect of suffering and death, perhaps the two most acute fears in life, he was desperately seeking respite. Krishna told him that running away from fear, or trying to artificially control the world to avoid fear, would ultimately prove futile. Deeper solutions are required.

Most people try to overcome fear through practical arrangements - an alarm on the house, health insurance for the family, abundant bank balance for the future and vaccinations for immunity. In addition we apply solutions on the mental level - things which alter our state of consciousness like drugs or affirmations. Some people seek intellectual solutions. They try to break fear down using logic, analysis and self-development wisdom. While all such attempts certainly provide some relief they don't get to the root of the problem.

In Chapter Eighteen Arjuna reaches the mature conclusion. He explains that his confusion, bewilderment and uncertainty has cleared. He has regained a vision for his life, and feels the inspiration and confidence to pursue it. He picks up his bow in determination, the same bow that was slipping from his hand in Chapter One. It was possible because Krishna expertly coached Arjuna in spiritual wisdom and recalibrated his vision of reality. Fear arises from misidentification with the temporary and disconnection from the spirit. Illumined spiritual consciousness empowers one to see every event, experience and emotion in the context of the bigger picture. Spiritualists live with the vision of eternity and are thus fully equipped to bring everything into perspective. They become sages of steady mind.

Srila Prabhupada was once asked what he feels when he chants Hare Krishna. His reply was interesting: *"I feel no fear!"* The greatest spiritualists didn't just philosophise about overcoming fear but powerfully demonstrated it through their own life. Srila Prabhupada suffered two heart attacks at sea, but never feared for his health. He came to America with 40 rupees, but never feared for his maintenance. He lived with drug addicts and hippies, but never feared for his safety. He renounced everything, but never feared for the future. Krishna thus invites everyone into this blissful, unbounded spiritual reality - *"Don't fear, don't hesitate, don't worry."*

"Arjuna said: My dear Krishna, O infallible one, my illusion is now gone. I have regained my memory by Your mercy. I am now firm and free from doubt and am prepared to act according to Your instructions."

(Bhagavad-gita 18.73)

References

18.30 – Real knowledge allows one to identify what is worthy of fear.

18.66 – Krishna reassures Arjuna there is no need for hesitation or worry.

Face your Fears

List the three most prominent fears in your life at present:

1.

2.

3.

1) What has caused them to become such big fears for you? Can you relate it to previous experiences or interactions? How did you 'learn' this fear?

2) How much does that fear limit your experience of life? What are you currently doing to deal with that fear?

3) How would spiritual wisdom and practice help you to overcome your fear? Do you have any experience of this happening in your life?

Now try to think of one practical thing you can start doing from tomorrow in order to overcome each fear.

Summary | How To

It's not coincidental that the Bhagavad-gita was spoken on a battlefield; an action-packed arena of intensity in which there is every complexity imaginable. Beware! The weight of the world can easily weigh you down. Take the empowering insights of these eighteen chapters and become fully equipped to expertly navigate the battlefield of life and emerge victorious. By employing these life hacks you won't just survive, but you'll thrive. The transformational power of the Bhagavad-gita can be experienced in the here and now.

Part Three: *Why Not?*

*The Bhagavad-gita refutes all the excuses
we may offer to delay our spiritual journey.*

	Excuse
1	"I don't have the time."
2	"I already know all of this."
3	"I have so many duties to fulfil."
4	"I'm not intelligent enough."
5	"I'd prefer to practically help the world."
6	"I'm too active – I just can't focus."
7	"I trust science and fact, not spirituality and faith."
8	"I'll do it in the future."
9	"I don't follow organised religion."
10	"I don't experience God – I've never seen Him."
11	"I have too many difficulties in my life."
12	"I'll lose all my friends."
13	"I'm already happy."
14	"I have too many bad habits."
15	"I'll lose my ambition and won't be successful."
16	"I see religion causes more problems."
17	"I've seen too much hypocrisy in religion."
18	"I don't want to be forced."

A man of unbreakable determination resolved to climb the peaks of the Himalayan ranges. After arriving at the foothills, he checked into his hotel room in preparation for the arduous expedition ahead. He rose the next morning, donned his mountaineering gear, and made his way to the hotel check out. Upon reaching the reception he peered outside and saw an aggressive snow storm in bitingly cold temperatures. Not a soul in sight. Undeterred and undaunted, he handed his keys to the receptionist and headed straight for the door. *"Where are you going?!"* the receptionist exclaimed, *"there's a weather warning and hazardous conditions – nobody treks in such a situation!"* Aware of the obvious obstacles, the trekker looked back with a sparkle in his eye and replied – *"Because my heart has already reached the peak, there won't be any problem for my body to reach."* With those prophetic words he ventured on, navigated the complexities and arrived at his desired destination.

If your heart reaches, everything else falls into place. When we have that determination, desire and rock-solid dedication, no external obstacle can disable our progress. If we're convinced, nothing can derail us. The Bhagavad-gita is an extraordinary book because it reveals the most adventurous, exciting and rewarding journey that anyone could possibly embark upon – a venture to the peaks of spiritual perfection where one comes face-to-face with God. It's the road less travelled, but the one which leads to the fulfilment of our innermost desire. If we implant the determination deep within, nothing can stop us - no excuse not to be successful.

In this section, we'll share with you eighteen everyday excuses that individuals often present to justify why they can't activate their spiritual journey. Upon close inspection, you'll see how Krishna, in each chapter of the Bhagavad-gita, ingeniously deconstructs every conceivable argument. He'll demonstrate that the only impediment to success is the compulsive tendency to disempower ourselves. Someone once told me – *"If you're good at making excuses then you'll never be good at anything else in your life!"* I witnessed their words of wisdom run true on more than one occasion!

How Krishna inspires Arjuna is truly poetry in motion. He doesn't just tell Arjuna what to do, but He educates him in *why* he should it and *how* he should do it. Further, Krishna's words instil an inspiration that empowers Arjuna to fully embrace the call to action. Sit back, open your heart, and let Krishna address every reservation. This is our chance to break free from the invisible chains that have impeded our spiritual growth for lifetimes.

" ❶ "

I don't have the
time

It's humbling to be on the receiving end of a sermon whilst being the speaker! At one event, an outspoken audience member asked me *"Are you married?"* I told him I wasn't. He challenged, *"Do you have a job?"* I told him I didn't. He inquired whether I ran a household and paid bills. Obviously not. He kept going, *"Do you have children?"* - it seemed so rhetorical I stayed silent. He triumphantly concluded that because I answered *"No"* to every question, I could say *"Yes"* to the prospect of spiritual development. I registered his line of thought - he was arguing that for those 'living in the world,' it's practically impossible to find quality time for spirituality.

Now it was my turn. Was Arjuna married? *Yes!* Did Arjuna have a host of worldly responsibilities? *Yes!* Was Arjuna running a household and looking after children? *Yes!* Did Arjuna have to contend with life complexities? *Yes!* Despite all these pressures, did Arjuna make time to reflect, introspect and question the direction of his life? *Yes!* Check mate!

Over 640 million soldiers had assembled on the battlefield of Kurukshetra, lined up like game pieces on a chess board. As the commanders manoeuvred the chariots into deadly formations, the atmosphere reached fever pitch. Everyone's adrenaline was pumping, and in the midst of it all stood Arjuna, the supreme archer, shouldering the heavyweight reputation of being the most formidable fighter of his time. All eyes were on him, watching with baited breath, wondering how he'd launch into battle and who he'd attack first.

At that moment, Arjuna did the unthinkable! He told Krishna to drive to the middle of the battlefield - not for strategic warfare purposes, but to step back, hit the pause button and contemplate his life direction.

It's impossible to capture the sheer unexpectedness of Arjuna's act! Despite being faced with practically every pressure under the sun to dive into action, Arjuna prioritised introspection. That takes incredible character. Can any of us say we're subjected to a more intense, chaotic or demanding situation than Arjuna? Seeing his predicament, can we complain that our life situation doesn't facilitate spiritual reflection? Saying we *"Don't have time"* for spirituality doesn't hold up. In life it's not about *having* time, it's about *making* time.

Imagine you embarked upon a car journey to Scotland, but never made the time to visit the petrol station to fuel up first? What if you were about to walk into an exam, but never made the time to attend the classes or revise the lessons? What if you took a pizza out of the freezer, but never made the time to heat it up in the oven? Some things are so crucial you have to make time. Failing to do so is not even an option. There's no escaping it.

Before we decide our goals in life, our direction, what we want to invest time, energy and resources into, we first need to understand who we are and what our purpose is in the grand scheme. Making time for this kind of questioning and spiritual realignment is not just a one-time affair. Every day is a battle, every day we're surrounded by intensity, every day we have to contend with obstacles, issues and dilemmas – and, therefore, every day we have to make time to remember the overarching purpose in the journey of life. Without that, we lose perspective.

"Arjuna said: O infallible one, please draw my chariot between the two armies so that I may see those present here, who desire to fight, and with whom I must contend in this great trial of arms."

(Bhagavad-gita 1.21-22)

References

1.20 – Arjuna decides to pause and reflect, which may have seemed like a weakness, but which brought complete clarity of vision.

Killing Time

In good time management, it's essential to distinguish between 'Urgent' and 'Important' activities. Herein, lies our main problem. 'Important' activities are the ones that will lead to ultimate (spiritual) success. These activities, however, don't necessarily demand and insist on your immediate, undivided attention. 'Urgent' activities are pressure points that need immediate resolution, though not necessarily contributing to the bigger picture.

The activities in Quadrant 1 are important, but they can end up dominating all of our time. The activities of Quadrants 3 and 4 are to be avoided as much as possible, or managed in indirect ways. This could involve reorganisation, delegation or minimisation. Effective people focus their time on Quadrant 2. Be careful not to mix up the urgent and the important.

	Urgent	Not Urgent
Important	*[Manage]* *do it now* Crisis Situation Emergency Medical Problem Family Issue Projects with deadlines Pressing problems	*plan for it* *[Focus]* Exercise Spiritual Development Planning Vocation Leisure / Relaxation Clarifying Values
Not Important	*[Avoid]* *delegate it* Certain Communication - emails, phone etc. Certain meetings & gatherings	*dump it* *[Avoid]* Trivial Tasks 'Escape' Activities Time Wasting Techniques Gossip

Assess the last week and categorise where the majority of your time is being spent. Are there any key activities that require a different approach?

" **2** **"**

I already
know all of this

Socrates famously said: *"My wisdom is that I know I don't know."* When we know very little we think we know a lot, and when we actually start exploring things deeply, we realise how much more there is to learn! Many people excuse themselves from spiritual pursuits thinking they know it all. *"I grew up with the Bhagavad-gita, it's been in my family for generations, my grandma used to tell me the stories when I was a kid – been there, done that, got the T-Shirt!"*

Arjuna was nurtured in a family of immaculate piety. He observed all customs and traditions, honoured *dharma* religiously, was guided by the most distinguished sages of the time, and had Krishna as his close companion. Despite this esteemed background, he humbly approached Krishna and conceded – *"I am confused, I have lost my composure – I am your disciple, please instruct me."* Of the assembled warriors, perhaps none were as qualified, successful, empowered and influential as Arjuna. Yet this formidable fighter opens himself up, in order to elevate himself higher.

Without the humility that Arjuna embodies there is no question of knowledge transmission - a proud person can't learn. In colloquial English we say they are *'full of it,'* a graphic term indicating that there's no space to insert anything fresh. Pride, and the stubbornness which accompanies it, blocks us from discovering, improving, transforming and evolving. Not only does pride create artificiality, but it maintains and breeds it. Despite having ample exposure to spiritual opportunities, proud people never really develop any substance.

Imagine all the knowledge in existence to be a large circle. One section represents *the things you know*. Another section represents *the things you know you don't know*. Interestingly, the biggest section is the third one, which represents *the things you don't know you don't know!* There is a wealth of knowledge in the world that we are completely oblivious to. Opening books like the Bhagavad-gita helps illuminate aspects of reality that we previously had no access to whatsoever. This is the most mysterious and fascinating part of the circle!

One of the biggest problems with modern education is that we tell people *what* to think rather than teaching them *how* to think. We're fed formulas and scripts, programmed to become bigger repositories of information, and systematically moulded to earn a living and rack up the numbers in the bank account. Yet if we were trained *how* to think, we would become explorers of wisdom, curious and hungry to grow, discover and venture into the unknown. We'd be equipped with the tools to realise our potential by going beyond the boundaries of what the world boxes us into.

Progressive life is a recurring venture into the unknown. In Chapter Ten, Krishna tells Arjuna that someone awakened to the spiritual reality is a *buddha*, an intelligent person. In the very next verse he says such persons eagerly come together and *enlighten* one another about Him! Enlightenment, then, is not a destination, but rather a direction. There is always more to learn about the unlimited spiritual dimension.

"Those who are seers of the truth have concluded that of the nonexistent [the material body] there is no endurance and of the eternal [the soul] there is no change. This they have concluded by studying the nature of both."

(Bhagavad-gita 2.16)

References

2.11 – Arjuna seemed to be speaking learned words, but was actually unaware of basic spiritual truths.

Library for Life

Of all his contributions, Srila Prabhupada's books are perhaps the most significant. His books have been read by people from all walks of life, translated into over eighty languages, and distributed in the millions. The meticulously translated writings constitute a veritable library of Vedic philosophy, religion, literature, and culture. Dr. Garry Gelade, a lecturer at Oxford University's Department of Philosophy, wrote of them: *"These texts are to be treasured. No one of whatever faith or philosophical persuasion who reads these books with an open mind can fail to be moved and impressed."*

Here is a rough guideline of how to progress through the library of Srila Prabhupada's books. You can tick them off as you complete them but remember that multipe readings bring deeper insights.

Srila Prabhupada's disciples and followers have also written and translated many valuable books which can enrich our understanding.

As with chanting, it's best to read daily, either a certain number of pages or for a certain amount of time. We can make a thorough study, noting interesting or difficult passages, or we can simply read our way through, confident of our spiritual edification. It's a good idea to offer respects to Krishna and His representatives before we begin reading. We can pray that the words we read will penetrate our heart and transform our character. Srila Prabhupada explains that besides reading, we should discuss spiritual topics with others. This is actually the best way to assimilate knowledge. There are courses at the temple and organised study groups in local areas.

Level	Outcomes	Books
1	Foundational philosophical understanding	Perfection of Yoga
		Chant and be Happy
		Perfect Questions Perfect Answers
		Raja Vidya: King of Knowledge
2	Detailed philosophical understanding	Science of Self Realisation
		Journey of Self Discovery
		Bhagavad-gita
		Sri Isopanisad
3	Practice of *bhakti-yoga*	Nectar of Instruction
		Nectar of Devotion
4	Relationship with Krishna & Srila Prabhupada	Krishna: The Supreme Personality of Godhead
		Prabhupada: Your Ever Well-wisher
5	Graduate Study	Teachings of Lord Caitanya
		Srimad-Bhagavatam
6	Post-graduate Study	Caitanya-Caritamrita

" 3 "

I have so many
duties to fulfil

Our lives are defined by multiple duties, responsibilities and roles to play. Faced with that pressure, we may naturally feel it more logical and practical to settle worldly demands first, free up some headspace, and then look to focus on spiritual development. A busy person may well conclude: *"Let me earn a little more money for security, let my kids grow up and settle down, let me tie up my business deals and secure a succession plan, let me pay off the remainder of my mortgage – after doing all this I'll surely dedicate myself to spiritual development."*

In Chapter Three, Krishna offers a more pragmatic solution by encouraging us to live a life of *integration*. He explains that material and spiritual duties are not sequential, such that when one set is complete we tackle the next. Rather, He explains that such duties should be synergised side-by-side. Krishna suggests that Arjuna fight as a warrior, and simultaneously cultivate his spiritual connection. Both must be balanced and appropriately factored into an integrated life. We're all playing multiple roles - as parents, children, workers, bosses, friends and leaders. People expect different things from us, and sometimes it feels as though the roles we play are conflicting. One demand seems to oppose another, time is limited, and if you make one person happy you seem to let someone else down. Damned if you do, damned if you don't!

Arjuna faced the same predicament. He had a *kula-dharma*, a duty to his family. He also had a *ksatriya-dharma*, a duty as a kingly warrior. Arjuna had a *pati-dharma*, a duty as a husband. Most importantly, Krishna reminded him about his *sanatana-dharma*, the *eternal* duty. When we invest time in building the foundation of *sanatana-dharma* in our life, it empowers us to fulfil everything else upon that steady platform. This brings all-round success. Krishna is not saying don't be a good husband, but rather become the best husband by being a *spiritual* husband. Krishna pushes Arjuna to fulfil his royal obligations by becoming a *spiritual* king. Krishna knows Arjuna's affection for the next generation and thus urges him to become a *spiritual* father.

Once, the saintly Narada Muni, famed for his spiritual acumen, encountered Vishnu. Ever-seeking improvement, he asked the Lord to identify the greatest devotee, to which Vishnu pointed out an unassuming farmer engaged in his daily work. Narada was shocked! Leaving aside the illustrious sages who had forsaken everything, here was a simple farmer being glorified as the greatest devotee! Vishnu promised to explain, but first gave Narada a bowl filled to the brim with oil, and told him to carry it around the universe and back... without spilling a drop! Narada set off, giving full attention to the task, and successfully returned without any spillages. When he triumphantly reported back the Lord asked him – *"While you were walking did you remember Me?"* Narada humbly admitted that the complex task of balancing the pot monopolised all his attention. The Lord pointed to the simple farmer – *"See how many things he is balancing – a job, a family and a host of other responsibilities, but in the midst of it constantly chants My names."* A humbling lesson. Integrated householders attract Krishna's attention by balancing many responsibilities and remaining ever alert to their spiritual duty.

"As the ignorant perform their duties with attachment to results, the learned may similarly act, but without attachment, for the sake of leading people on the right path."

(Bhagavad-gita 3.25)

References

3.4 – Prematurely giving up the world won't be beneficial in spiritual development.

3.8 – The discharge of essential duties facilitate physical maintenance and spiritual elevation.

Work as Worship

Our occupation can often seem an obstacle to progressive spirituality. The competitive climate, stressful lifestyle and weighty responsibilities can create frustration and confusion as we pursue our spiritual aspirations. Is it possible to operate in this dog-eat-dog world and still maintain our spirituality? Can one serve God via their worldly profession? The Bhagavad-gita offers the '3R' formula on how to spiritualise your daily work.

Consider your daily work in the world – is there a way you could incorporate these three elements in a more powerful way so as to spiritualise your occupation?

Righteous – First, one must endeavour to engage in righteous work. Certain occupations and livelihoods are based on exploitation, violence, dishonesty, and generally cause harm and disruption in the world. Such work is neither progressive for the individual nor prosperous for society at large. Although every type of work in today's world is tainted by some fault or imperfection, the spiritualist should nevertheless strive for a career that promotes harmony, compassion and upliftment.

Results – Second, we can dedicate the 'fruits' of our work to God. Such fruits come in the form of remuneration, knowledge, expertise, skills and influence in a particular field. Some measure of wealth is required to survive in the world, providing the necessities of food, clothing and shelter, but a certain portion should be reserved for spiritual causes. By offering charitable contributions towards the worship of Krishna and the spiritual upliftment of others, one also develops detachment and selflessness, which are the key ingredients in the spiritual journey.

Remembrance – Third, one should cultivate an active spiritual consciousness of Krishna while at work. Newly-wedded couples are wrapped in thoughts of each other even when separated and otherwise occupied. Eventually, our remembrance of Krishna will be just as natural. In the meantime we can make a conscious effort; keep devotional pictures on your desk, set computer passwords to Krishna's names, talk to your colleagues about spirituality, play spiritual music in the background... be imaginative! We must perform our daily duties with due care and attention, but actively remember that we are ultimately working for Krishna, our true employer and master.

" ④ **"**

I'm not
intelligent enough

When the lights go off we become blind, but when the lights turn on many hours later, the glaring effulgence can blind us in a different way! People sometimes feel like that when they approach spiritual literature. The volume of information, depth of the concepts and intricacy of the language can seem beyond our comprehension. *"I don't know Sanskrit, I'm not a philosopher, I'm not even a reader,"* someone may say, *"so what hope is there for me?"* For many people, when it comes to spiritual discourses, the knowledge goes in one ear and out the other. *Can this advanced theology actually be grasped by anyone and everyone?*

In Chapter Four, entitled "Transcendental Knowledge," this reservation is directly addressed. Krishna highlights how profound this wisdom is, and goes on to outline the qualification to fully grasp it. Interestingly, it's nothing to do with one's intellectual or analytical ability, but more to do with sincerity and devotion. Krishna reassures Arjuna: *"You can enter into the mysteries of this spiritual science, because you are My friend and My devotee."*

One need not be a scholar, scientist or philosophical genius, and sometimes being so can actually become counter-productive! One simply has to have a sincere and willing heart, genuinely seeking spiritual connection and a divine interaction with Krishna. The Bhagavad-gita is knowledge which is understood in the recesses of the heart, not simply within the brain. When we have a deep desire to understand and a seriousness to actually apply it in our life, then one is supplied with the necessary intelligence to grasp it.

Krishna further delineates the specific methodology by which this knowledge is accessed. One must first approach a spiritual teacher and inquire from them in all humility. Beyond passive listening, Krishna encourages one to then present thoughtful questions before that person to clarify their understanding and learn the nuanced application. Furthermore, the transmission of knowledge should include a practical demonstration of one's gratitude and dedication to their teacher. Humble listening, thoughtful questioning and heartfelt service – the three indispensable ingredients in the science of spiritual learning.

The knowledge of spiritual life is not just about acquiring more and more information. Sometimes people consider the process of education to be linear - learning more and more and more. More verses, more stories and more philosophy. Spiritual learning, however, is more like a spiral – you hear the same verses, the same stories, the same philosophical passages, but study them from different angles of vision and gradually home in on the essence of the message. Fundamental spiritual truths, simple but profound, are integrated within our consciousness and act to illumine our lives.

The essence of the Bhagavad-gita is actually very simple; we are spiritual beings, God is the supreme spirit, and when we give our heart to Him in a selfless, unmotivated way then not only do we rediscover our love for Krishna, but we awaken our love for everyone and everything around us. We rediscover our love for life.

"That very ancient science of the relationship with the Supreme is today told by Me to you because you are My devotee as well as My friend and can therefore understand the transcendental mystery of this science."

(Bhagavad-gita 4.3)

References

4.34 – The science of learning from a spiritual master.

4.35 – The result of cultivating knowledge through this methodology.

Walk the Talk

Consider the following statements, which encapsulate some fundamental teachings of the Bhagavad-gita. Now identify behaviours and observations in your life that demonstrate you may not have fully internalised these statements. Can you think of a few changes to your life that may help you to further apply these statements in reality?

	Behaviours which indicate I haven't fully internalised this	What could I do to bring this philosophy into reality?
"We are not the body, we are the soul"		
"Everything we experience is happening under divine providence and meant for our ultimate wellbeing"		
"Pursuing selfish sense gratification leads to misery"		
"We are not in control of the results of our activities, but can only endeavour to the best of our ability"		
"If we live by the wisdom of scripture our lives will be happier, healthier and more spiritually successful"		

Pick a random purport from the Bhagavad-gita (e.g. 2.7), and go point-by-point noting down your responses to the two questions above.

5

I'd prefer to practically help the world

2020 was one of the most challenging years in the history of the world - a global pandemic that brought practically every part of the world to its knees. Scenes of suffering confront us every day, and we feel impelled to be an agent of positive change. *What can spirituality really do to help? One may worship, pray and chant but isn't it more important to do something practical and tangible to help the world? Wouldn't time, energy and resource be better spent in hands-on welfare work rather than ethereal meditation? How can spirituality address the environmental, economic, political and social problems facing our generation? Isn't it selfish to focus on cultivating our own spirituality, rather than selflessly helping others?*

In a beautiful verse from Chapter Five, Krishna explains how those endowed with knowledge and gentleness (*vidya vinaya*) naturally become spiritually realised (*pandita*), causing their vision to become universal (*sama darsinah*). This spiritual vision enables them to see the equality of all living beings beyond external difference, and the divinity in all aspects of creation. It is this elevation of consciousness that's the greatest need of the day.

For a moment, consider the problems that surround us and try to decipher the root cause. A closer inspection reveals that most of them stem from a lack of spiritual vision. Some people are programmed to exploit, pillage and hoard, whereas others will nurture, share and give. Some people make every decision in life based on how it facilitates their enjoyment and pleasure, while others have a broader vision which considers beyond their own instant gratification. Are we driven by selfishness, or has selflessness become second nature? The answers to these questions reveal our vision on the continuum of material to spiritual. The fundamental cause behind every issue in the world is a severe lack of spiritual vision – racism, sexism, nationalism, ageism – all based on the body, which is just a temporary, superficial covering of the spirit self.

During the British rule of India, the government was concerned about the number of venomous cobra snakes in Delhi. To mitigate the issue, the Government advertised a generous bounty for every dead cobra. The strategy met with immediate success as large numbers of snakes were killed for the reward. Later, however, enterprising people began to breed cobras and then turn them over for the extra income. When the Government realised what had happened they scrapped the scheme. The cobra-breeders then set all the 'worthless' snakes free, and the number of cobras increased exponentially! Not only do artificial solutions fail to address the root cause, but they often aggravate the problem due to ignorance of the unintended consequences of the so-called solution.

Though we're all eager to jump into action and do something to improve the world, it's worthwhile spending some time to develop our spiritual vision and deeply understand how to help the situation. We need to solve the immediate problems but also prevent them from resurfacing. We need solutions which are comprehensive and sustainable. The passion to serve the world must be guided by a compass of knowledge, because when that passion meets the compass, then it becomes true compassion.

"The humble sages, by virtue of true knowledge, see with equal vision a learned and gentle brahmana, a cow, an elephant, a dog and a dog-eater [outcaste]."

(Bhagavad-gita 5.18)

News of the World

The principles of the Bhagavad-gita are versatile enough to apply in any given situation. Read the following iconic newspaper headlines and consider how you would give a spiritual perspective on them based on the Gita's teachings. What would be your diagnosis and recommendation?

'The Titanic Sinks' [16th April 1912] - Journalists were still in denial that a ship thought to be unsinkable could have failed so catastrophically.

'Greatest Crash in Wall Street's History' [25th October 1929] - The economic crash of 1929, fuelled by uncertainty following an artificial share price boom, was the worst in U.S. history. On 24th October, panicked investors traded an astonishing 12.9 million shares.

'Beatle John Lennon Slain' *[9th December 1980]* - At 10.49pm, John Lennon was shot in the back four times by Mark David Chapman, a fan who had been stalking him for 3 months.

'War on America' *[12th September 2001]* - On 11th September 2001, terrorists hijacked four commercial passenger jet airliners, crashing two of them into the Twin Towers and a third into the Pentagon.

'Indonesian Tsunami' *[28th December 2004]* - Just after midnight on 26th December 2004, an earthquake off the west coast of Sumatra, Indonesia, triggered a huge tsunami, which killed over 225,000 people in 11 countries.

" **6** "

I'm too active –
I just can't focus

The complexity of modern civilisation is mind-boggling, causing us all, monks included, to complicate our lives in order to keep up. It's a far cry from the villages of bygone ages where people moved much slower and spiritual culture was woven into the fabric of day-to-day life. The chaotic environment relentlessly bombards our consciousness, generating a myriad of agitations and provocations. *"I'll never be able to spiritually connect,"* some people say, *"I'm too energetic, active, and restless – I struggle to sit quietly for even five minutes!"*

Arjuna is on the same page as us, while Krishna is one step ahead. In Chapter Six, the consummate warrior, equipped to battle anyone or anything, admits his powerlessness in contending with his own formidable mind. He says his mind is uncontrollably flickering (*cancalam*), agitated (*pramarthi*), powerful (*balavad*) and stubborn (*drdham*). *"To control the mind,"* Arjuna concludes, *"is more difficult than controlling the wind!"* Most of us living in the urban jungle are faced with the same predicament.

Some posit that meditation is out of the question, though in reality it's an indispensable necessity! We need to revisit the logic. You don't cure your disease and *then* go to the hospital. You don't fill your belly and *then* visit a restaurant. You don't get fit and *then* signup to the gym. These places and activities are actually there to help you achieve your goal! In the same way, the reason we factor in spiritual stillness, sometimes forcibly, is because it's the only way to cure our chronic restlessness. If someone comes to me and says *"My life is so chaotic that I can't meditate for even ten minutes,"* then I look at them and reply, *"For you, meditation is prescribed for* twenty *minutes!"*

Krishna is not suggesting we turn away from being active, energetic and driven. He instead recommends that we direct our energies in the most effective and efficient way, and to do that requires scheduled times of non-activity and contemplation. An archer's goal is to hit the target as quick and powerfully as possible. Ironically, the first movement is to pull the arrow *away* from the target. It may seem antithetical, but that backward motion allows one to generate more power, pinpoint the aim, and seize the most opportune moment to unleash the energy.

When we sit down to meditate, a million thoughts may whizz through the mind, impelling us to jump into action! There may be doubts and uncertainties about situations, friction in relationships, worries and concerns about issues, excitement and anticipation about future opportunities. The mind is a busy place!

We remind ourselves that everything in life is perfectly resolved by deepening our spirituality. The problem is not other people – it's often our own lack of tolerance, empathy and sensitivity. The problem is not the situation that surrounds us – it's our inner rigidity, stubbornness and lack of broader vision. All our aspirations and dreams can be fulfilled beyond our wildest imagination, but only after we fine tune our motivations and shelve our selfish agendas. Everything is achieved through spiritual purity, and spiritual purity comes from determined, focused spiritual practice. After we meditate, perspectives change, and life looks much different.

"A transcendentalist should always engage his body, mind and self in relationship with the Supreme; he should live alone in a secluded place and should always carefully control his mind. He should be free from desires and feelings of possessiveness."

(Bhagavad-gita 6.10)

References

6.36 – Yoga practice and mental control must go hand in hand.

The Yoga of Writing

One of the most effective ways to better understand your mind, its movements, and how to remould it, is through the powerful process of journaling. Words are not just a means of expressing ourselves, but a way to discover ourselves.

Broadly speaking, we could say there are two aspects of the self:

Impulsive self – the senses and mind, which instinctively respond to the stimuli of the world.

Reflective self – the intelligence and soul, which are empowered with insight and discrimination.

Journaling facilitates an interaction between the two so we can harness the benefits of both.

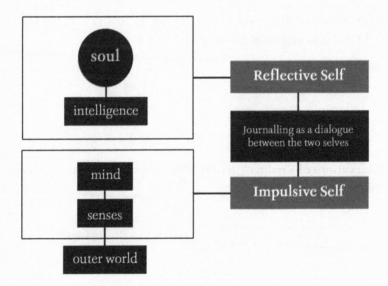

In your journal reflect on the following observations through the lens of scriptural wisdom. As an experiment reflect on this week:

Observations of the day – the lessons learnt from conversations, interactions and events of the day.

Observations of oneself – analysis of one's own lifestyle, character, attitude, and general response to various situations.

Observations of the world – reflecting on the affairs of the material world and how various environments affect us.

Observations of Krishna – detecting the messages, interventions and arrangements of Krishna within our life.

7

I trust science & fact, not spirituality & faith

Many spiritual practitioners have a simple-heartedness which allows them to naturally invest themselves in the path. Some may look down upon that as naïve and sentimental, while others may wish they had the same in order to quieten the 'inner sceptic.' To a greater or lesser extent, each of us do have a need for evidence and empirical backup – hard facts for the head that allow for an investment of the soft heart.

In Chapter Seven, Krishna highlights the proposition of Bhagavad-gita as more of a spiritual science than a sectarian faith. In the very first verse He stresses the absolute necessity of hearing spiritual insight (*tac chrnu*). The aural reception of knowledge descending from a higher source may seem counter-intuitive to scientific discovery, but that's not entirely true. The process begins with hearing, but it matures into a direct perception of the self (*pratyaksa vagamam*). On this path of spiritual science we discover there are no HOLES in its efficacy:

H – Hear - first we broaden our horizons and expand our field of discovery by hearing from a source which is beyond our inherently limited sphere of understanding.

O – Observe - we verify those paradigms by comparing them with our own observations – of ourselves, of people around us, and of the world in general.

L – Live – when things tally, it bolsters our faith and we feel inspired to apply many of the principles in our day-to-day functioning – we bring spirituality into the 'lab of life.'

E – Experience – that application triggers tangible spiritual experience and helps us progress beyond a mere philosophical and intellectual engagement with God.

S – Share – the personal revelation impels one to share it with others, and this compassionate, selfless dissemination brings heightened experiences of the spiritual reality.

Conventional religious discourse, as presented today, begins with belief and ends in belief. If people interface with the Bhagavad-gita in the same way, it will also remain a belief. If, however, one is ready to seriously engage with the spiritual experiment offered in the pages of the Bhagavad-gita, then one unearths an actual experience, observation and realisation of the spiritual reality. This is the most wondrous scientific experiment in the entire universe - the experiment to find our true self.

The Gita doesn't propose anything less scientific than what we see in mainstream empiricism. When we take a closer look at what is headlined as irrevocable scientific fact, we'll see there is much more to the story – substantial underlying faith, irrational resistance to opposing evidence, and superficial hype and claims of discovery far beyond what has actually been unearthed. Science is not as factual as we may think, and spirituality is not as faith-based as many automatically (and dogmatically) conclude. When you apply the same level of scrutiny to science and spirituality you'll see that it's somewhat of a level playing field. *Which experiment will you take?*

"I shall now declare unto you in full this knowledge, both phenomenal and numinous. This being known, nothing further shall remain for you to know."

(Bhagavad-gita 7.2)

References

7.2 – Hearing from spiritual sources gives insights into all aspects of reality.

7.3 – Realisation of the Supreme Lord is rare, and is achieved through transformation of consciousness.

Faith Issues

It's clear that faith is very much a part of life. We required faith to begin an educational endeavour, to build a relationship, to travel from one country to another - faith is embedded within every aspect of life, and without it we'd be rendered dysfunctional.

Can you pinpoint three prominent reservations which impede your wholehearted investment of faith in the wisdom of the Gita? Explore why these doubts may have arisen within you, and what the underlying causes may be. What could be the solution to overcome these blocks and open the path to greater spiritual experience?

Why is it difficult to invest my faith in Bhagavad-gita and the spiritual process?	What may be the deeper, underlying causes of this?	What could I do to overcome these blocks and more wholeheartedly give myself?

❝ **8** ❞
I'll do it
in the future

'Tomorrow' is a mystical land where 99% of human creativity, potential and achievement lies. Unfortunately, 99% of people never enter that space! We have an annoying tendency to put things off, even when we know they're valuable, desirable and doable. A heavy inertia grounds us into stagnation and we're not able to seize the day – not because there are practical or perceived obstacles, but simply because we fall victim to laziness and procrastination.

In Chapter Eight, Krishna highlights the ultimate meditation to reinstate clarity into every aspect of our lives. He reminds Arjuna that this body is a ticking time bomb, a fact that hasn't fully registered with most people. When it comes to spirituality, the teenagers say *"I'm too young,"* the elderly say *"I'm too old,"* and everyone in between says *"I'm too busy!"* They say they'll do it *"Someday."* The irony is that there are seven days in a week and *"Someday"* is not one of them! If our mentality is *"I'll do it tomorrow"* then tomorrow our answer may well remain *"I'll do it tomorrow!"* Thus we circle the cycle, life after life.

It's a dangerous approach. The pain of discipline is uncomfortable but the pain of regret is unbearable. If we fail to wholeheartedly dedicate ourselves to doing what we know is ultimately valuable, we'll find it hard to forgive ourselves down the line. Krishna reminds us that before time runs out, we must ensure our spiritual consciousness has blossomed. Indeed, our hopes, concerns and desires in those final moments will determine our next destination.

Spiritual success doesn't magically appear overnight, like an apple that randomly drops from a tree and mystically hits you. Spiritual success comes in instalments every single day, and when we apply ourselves to the process on any given day, we receive the instalment of success set aside for that day. If we procrastinate and put off, we lose out. Every single day, for the rest of our lives, we have the opportunity to keep investing in that eternal account. After all, that final balance will trigger our thoughts at the time of death.

We can also up the stakes. Higher investments mean higher risk. Throughout history, we see how distinguished saints pushed the barriers of their comfort zone, embraced uncertainty, and voluntarily accepted precarious situations in pursuit of their purpose. I'm not sure whether they began with concrete conviction, but they certainly ended up with it! It spurred their dependence upon the will of providence. Token religious faith is commendable, but life becomes dynamically exciting when we experience the mystery and wonder of divine intervention. Selfless sacrifices, exceptional endeavours and the willingness to take a risk are the drivers behind such experiences. How can we connect with the hand of God if we don't have the courage to let go of the perpetual pursuance of comfort, convenience and control?

It's easy to gravitate towards the 'safe options' in life. Don't do anything drastic, tread the path of least resistance and keep things sweet and simple. The world has its preconceived notions – what's acceptable and what's not – and we just fit right in. The fear of embarrassment, failure and public scrutiny is too much, and thus plagued by the disease of conformity, we perpetually confine and limit ourselves. Yet a comfortable life is itself a hazardous disease. With it comes the danger of mechanical, ritualistic, mediocre, and stagnated spirituality. In the name of caution, we sell ourselves short.

"For one who always remembers Me without deviation, I am easy to obtain, O son of Prtha, because of his constant engagement in devotional service."

(Bhagavad-gita 8.14)

References

8.28 – By developing one's devotion, the results of all other pious and religious processes automatically come about.

Enemies of Growth

With each day comes the opportunity to grow. Amongst the plethora of factors which stagnate spiritual growth, three stand prominent. We slide into mediocrity and averageness when we're too busy, too arrogant or too comfortable to invest in our life.

Reflect on the three ingredients of growth below. What are your blocks to growth and how can you overcome them? What tangible changes can you make immediately?

Time – our valuable hours are consumed by pressing issues and daily demands. Some things surely require immediate attention, but we have a chronic tendency to unnecessarily promote tasks in our 'to-do list' that may well be urgent but not really very important. Thus, we end up neglecting that which doesn't frantically tag on our consciousness, but which is key to the bright future ahead – time spent reflecting, planning, challenging and questioning. We need to free up quality time and mental space to 'think out of the box.'

Humility – to improve, we must first acknowledge that we're not the best version of ourselves. This requires humility. We think often ourselves one step ahead of everyone else, and our own pride blocks us from seeing how we could be wrong. A humble person accepts their limitations, looks for guidance, ever seeking an opportunity to refine and enhance their character and lifestyle.

Courage – life is a perennial tension between comfort and aspiration. We seek to explore, to grow, to achieve, yet we also desire security, safety and certainty. Truth be told, we have to sacrifice one to get the other. If we opt to remain in the comfort-zone, we may have to live with the inevitable feelings of an unexciting and lifeless existence. On the other hand, if we dive for our dreams we'll have to ready ourselves to brave the rocky road of uncertainty and obstacle. Every significant achievement has its price tag. In an age where security, establishment and balanced prosperity have become the guiding beacons for our comfortable life, only a few have the courage to follow their dreams.

9

I don't follow
organised religion

A saintly person floated forward with a shining halo around his head and when asked what mission he was on, he replied, *"I'm starting a spiritual movement."* Following closely behind was the devil, and when quizzed about his intention, he replied *"I'll be helping him to organise it!"*

Who can deny the potentiality of pure spirituality being side-lined in the sticky matrix of organised religion? The institution can become about superiority over humility. We may stress the afterlife, but forget about the here-life. Rules and regulations take prominence, sometimes at the expense of individual expression. Meetings over relationships, numbers over faces, holiness over humanity, monologue over dialogue, doctrine over character, appearance over authenticity – the pitfalls are endless! Many people thus resolve to distance themselves from organised religion, opting to pursue spiritual awakening in their own private arena.

Krishna fully endorses the notion of heartfelt spirituality. In Chapter Nine, He emphatically asserts that no matter how simple an external spiritual offering may be, a single leaf, fruit or flower, if it's offered with sincere devotion and purity of consciousness, it becomes irresistibly attractive. In the very next verse, however, Krishna states: *"Whatever you do, whatever you eat, whatever you offer or give away, and whatever austerities you perform—do that, O Arjuna, as an offering to Me."* Spirituality is undoubtedly an affair of the heart, but in order to awaken that natural and spontaneous devotion we require a systemised regime of dedication.

If someone wanted to express their heart through music, but never learnt notes and keys, how much would they be able to express? If someone wanted to express their heart through writing, but never took the time to learn spelling and grammar, how much would they be able to express? If someone wanted to express their heart through spirituality, but they never took the time to engage in spiritual practice (*sadhana*), would there really be any genuine awakening? The regulated practice of spirituality helps us to overcome the ignorance, imperfection and inner blocks that impede the free-flowing expression of our innate devotion.

Srila Prabhupada established a house in which the whole world can live. The vision was to give every individual unlimited opportunities, facilities and support to powerfully engage in acts of devotion. The essence is to bring together sincere spiritual seekers so they can inspire and empower each other. After all, those who embark on the journey towards transcendence are brave indeed. They strive for purity in a world of degradation, embrace simplicity amongst rampant materialism, and cultivate selflessness in an atmosphere charged with exploitation. As we swim upstream, we'll undoubtedly be faced with temptation, doubt, ridicule and moments of weakness. The support of spiritual friends is an indispensable ingredient in spiritual success.

Our individual spiritual lives are like a boat, and the organised institution is like a river. If we ride that water and interact appropriately, it carries us to our destination. If that water hijacks the boat and enters within, however, we drown all the way down. The institution is not the essence, but it is essential. Everyone can experience the benefits of it in their spiritual journey.

"Engage your mind always in thinking of Me, become My devotee, offer obeisances to Me and worship Me. Being completely absorbed in Me, surely you will come to Me."

(Bhagavad-gita 9.34)

References

9.27 – How to connect every aspect of life to the spiritual goal.

9.28 – Spiritual connection frees one from karma.

Mechanics of Spirituality

At 4.30am each morning the monks commence their 4-hour spiritual workout – a dedicated regime, 365 days a year. To an onlooker it may seem monotonous and mechanical; a holy 'boot camp.' Seasoned spiritualists, however, will testify that these tried and tested practices open up an internal world of bottomless depth. As we progressively upgrade the quality, becoming more conscious, attuned and reflective, fresh and new experiences surface. Spiritual tools are timeless and limitless.

Yet the mechanics of spirituality can also degenerate into a monotonous ritual. When we neglect to invest our heart in these simple acts of devotion, we start tending towards being dogmatically religious rather than dynamically spiritual. Here are some classic symptoms of mechanical spirituality:

- I 'fit in' my practices as opposed to prioritising a suitable time of day.

- I 'multi-task' my practices as opposed to giving them exclusive focus and attention.

- I have no serious plans (or desires) to increase and enhance my practices.

- I look for excuses and justification to neglect my spiritual practices.

- I lack quality remembrance of the goal and purpose while performing my spiritual practices.

- The mind frequently wanders during my practices, and I happily let it travel.

Would you answer 'yes' to any of the above? Why may this situation have arisen, and what can you do to rectify it?

❝ **10** **❞**

I don't experience God – I've never seen Him

I once met a lady who expressed frustration in her attempts to find God. She told me her story: two years of spiritual travels, countless nights of prayer, diligent scriptural exploration and regular introspection, but still no sign! *"Will I ever find Him?"* she asked. *"I'm beginning to question whether He even exists."* What to speak of the 'searchers', even the faithful often doubt that their Supreme friend is actually alive, alert and active. A seeming lack of reciprocation and intervention can discourage even the most dedicated spiritualist. *Where is God when you need Him? Can we commit ourselves to a person we've never really directly interacted with?*

In Chapter Ten, Krishna demonstrates how He is fully available for anyone who wants to perceive His presence. In a celebrated verse He explains how all beautiful, breath-taking and bountiful creations of the world are but a spark of His splendour. Krishna says He is the taste of water, the light of the sun and moon, the sound in ether and the ability in every person. *Does a day go by without drinking water, seeing the luminaries in the sky, experiencing the silence around us and meeting gifted people?*

God is fully available, but the question is whether *we're* awake and alert.

Whilst at university, I was obliged to read several books on effective management. As I browsed some old notes an interesting quote caught my attention: *"The best managers create systems and inspire people, thus you don't even see them and you don't even know they're there."* By their ingenuity, everything inconspicuously works like a dream. When Krishna explains how He manages the entire cosmos, He cites the analogy of a necklace. All universal affairs are actually resting upon Him, He says, just as pearls are strung upon a thread. The thread is the essential binding factor, giving the necklace its form and shape. Interestingly, however, the thread remains entirely invisible to our eyes.

People yearn for a direct experience and perception of things. The fact that we cannot see God at work, that He hasn't appeared in person before our eyes, relating to us face-to-face, seems to be a major sticking point. *"Show me God, and then I'll believe in Him,"* the sceptics posit. Even according to the management gurus of the 21st century, however, God would be a pretty average manager if He was frantically running around in front of us directing everything.

If you look at the top CEOs in the modern business world, they setup a managerial hierarchy and then take a back seat, allowing things to function effortlessly without their direct day-to-day involvement. You'll probably find them relaxing at the golf course with their friends. Thus, the fact that we can't see God creating and maintaining this universe may not be a disqualification, but rather credit to His expert organisational proficiency. He manages the material universes through others, and frees up His quality time to intimately relate with His loving devotees in the spiritual world.

"Of all creations I am the beginning and the end and also the middle, O Arjuna. Of all sciences I am the spiritual science of the self, and among logicians I am the conclusive truth."

(Bhagavad-gita 10.32)

References

10.16 – Arjuna inquires as to how Krishna can be perceived in the opulence of this world.

10.17-42 – Krishna describes how one can actually think about Him, meditate on Him and see Him everywhere.

Time for God

Until we have that face-to-face interaction with Krishna, there are other immediate ways to contact Him. God is transcendent (beyond this world) and simultaneously immanent (perceivable in our immediate realm). One can perceive His presence in the following ways, though it does require a quality investment of TIME to forge that connection:

T - Temple Deity - God's immanence in the material world may be brought to perception when material elements, such as marble, metal or wood, become sacred forms of worship according to authorised prescriptions.

I - Individual Beings - Krishna explains He is within the hearts of all living beings and from Him comes knowledge, remembrance and forgetfulness. We can interact with Him through others.

M - Material Nature - while God is the source of the universe, He is simultaneously present within it. Indeed, He declares in Bhagavad-gita that whatever wondrous and beautiful creations we see, spring from but a spark of His splendour.

E - Events of Life - we may not see God's face, but we can perceive His hand in everyday events and experiences. By fine-tuning our consciousness, we can begin to perceive the dynamic ways in which Krishna intervenes in our lives and crafts beautiful arrangements.

Can you think of instances where you feel you have encountered God in these ways? What convinces you it was something spiritual and not just your mind?

" 11 "

I have too many
difficulties in my life

Over twenty years ago, after graduating from UCL (University College London) with a Bachelor's degree, I opted out of the 'suit and tie' corporate world and adopted the robes of monasticism instead. Ironically, it's all come full circle; dealing with people, projects and practicalities is an inescapable part of life. This monk must have some management karma to burn off! The reality is that whoever you are and whatever your situation may be, life is full of inescapable difficulty - financial problems, family problems, career problems, relationship problems, problems, problems and more problems! In the midst of it all, how do we find the headspace to embrace spirituality with focus, optimism and determination?

Consider the problems that Arjuna encountered in his life. When he was young he lost his father, and later was subjected to severe mistreatment and exploitation from his own family members. He and his brothers experienced injustice and insult, their kingdom usurped, harshly stripped of their entire identity. It all reaches a climax when Arjuna faces the biggest obstacle of his life so far - the prospect of battle and bloodshed with his near and dear ones. A rollercoaster journey to say the least. If anyone was entitled to lodge a complaint about being dealt a bad hand, the Pandava brothers would probably top the list.

In Chapter Eleven, Krishna expertly allays Arjuna's concerns by displaying His inconceivable feature known as the Universal Form. Within it, Arjuna witnesses the entirety of creation, all the planets, demigods and living entities, and the entire sequence of past, present and future. When Arjuna peered into this extraordinary display he saw all of his adversaries meeting their death, even though the battle had not even begun. Krishna poignantly told Arjuna that all of his enemies and obstacles had already been annihilated by the will of providence and his only task was to become an instrument in the plan.

The reversals of this world, Krishna says, flow in and out of our life like the cosmic seasons. Some periods are harsh and challenging, yet they have their part to play in the grand scheme of things. Spiritual practice won't necessarily make all the problems disappear, but it will empower you with elevated spiritual vision and an inner immunity come what may. The problem is not the problem. The problem is our reaction to the problem. Instead of waiting for a peaceful situation around us, the greatest need of the day is to create a peaceful situation within us.

There were two boys who had an alcoholic father. One of them became an alcoholic while the other stayed away for his entire life. The alcoholic son was asked why he succumbed to this habit. He answered: *"My whole childhood I watched my alcoholic father."* The other son was asked why he took the route of abstention. His answer: *"My whole childhood I watched my alcoholic father."* Ironic! Subjected to the same problem, but influenced in opposite ways. The challenge is to become like water, effortlessly flowing around any obstructing rocks and moving steadily to the destination. The Bhagavad-gita trains the avid student to reside in their sacred space, never allowing their inner world to be hijacked by the chaos of life.

"As the many waves of the rivers flow into the ocean, so do all these great warriors enter into Your blazing mouths."

(Bhagavad-gita 11.28)

References

11.36 – Whatever Krishna does is always for the ultimate good.

Digesting Life

When challenging situations arise in life, here are four powerful questions you can ask yourself which will help to frame the situation and give hope, inspiration and growth:

- Is it personal? – *Was it really about me?*

- Is it permanent? – *Will it pass?*

- Is it pervasive? – *Does it affect my whole life or just a part of it?*

- Is it potentially positive? – *Can it offer me some unique opportunity to develop?*

Think of a time when you experienced a set back and a door closed on you. What doors subsequently opened? What can you do to notice new doors opening?

" 12 "

I will lose
all of my friends

When we embrace spirituality our entire worldview shifts, causing our habits, goals and interests to subsequently change. It's inevitable that the relationships with people who we shared so much with will also change. It can be unsettling on both sides, and we may fear losing our friends and family forever, wondering whether that emotional gap can ever be filled. *Can spirituality alienate us from the society we live in and cause us to lose our friends?*

In Chapter Twelve, Krishna describes how the awakening of pure devotion upgrades one's character in a beautiful way. One who sincerely and seriously takes to spiritual life frees themselves from envy (*advesta*), becomes friendly and compassionate to all (*maitrah karuna*), gives up all sense of greed and proprietorship (*nirmamo*), and is purified of pride, arrogance and vanity (*nirahankarah*). In all situations the devotee embodies equanimity, and remains unaffected by the inevitable rollercoaster journey of life (*sama dukkha sukha ksami*).

Far from losing friends, with genuine spiritual advancement comes the increased capability to have gracious relationships with one and all. Equipped with spiritual vision that penetrates beyond the externals, one remains unaffected by annoying idiosyncrasies, ideological differences, unpredictable personalities, and undesirable character traits. We're able to see something deeper, the underlying beauty of the spirit. We can see the heart. At this stage of purity, we have no enemies, even if others view us as such. When we become spiritually immersed, we actually find real friendships, and also become real friends to others.

The metaphor of a tree can help us better understand our interactions in this world. Some friends are like *leaves* – they come and go, changing with the winds and seasons, in our life for a few scenes of the story. They appear beautiful, but the next moment they disappear. Other friends are like *branches* - they're stronger, stay for longer and foster a greater confidence and reliance within us. At some point, however, they also snap and turn out to be unpredictable. These friendships, which we strongly identify with, lack the deep substance of genuine connection. A few rare friendships are like the trunk, which stay for the entirety of one's lifetime and provide constant support and nourishment in our life. Those friends, often overlooked, are solid and substantial. They accept us for who we are. Through this lens we can better understand the varieties of friendship, and become better equipped to ascertain where it genuinely exists in our life.

In concluding Chapter Twelve, Krishna expresses how he becomes conquered by those who wholeheartedly invest themselves in the process of loving devotion, *bhakti-yoga*. On the spiritual journey one is ultimately introduced to the best friend of all – Krishna! Through that relationship with Krishna, our connection with everyone else naturally blossoms. When we shine a light into a diamond, that light is beautifully reflected in all directions. Similarly, when we direct our friendship toward Krishna, the diamond, that mood of fraternity expands unlimitedly.

"One who is not envious but is a kind friend to all living entities, who does not think himself a proprietor and is free from false ego, who is equal in both happiness and distress, who is tolerant, always satisfied, self-controlled, and engaged in devotional service with determination, his mind and intelligence fixed on Me – such a devotee of Mine is very dear to Me."
(Bhagavad-gita 12.13-14)

References

12.13-14 – The friendly nature of the spiritualist that also connects them with the Supreme Friend.

Best Friends

Real friends have three principle qualities – they resonate with your personality (*sajatiya*), have genuine feelings of affection for you (*snehasya*), and are actually able to help you because of their maturity and wisdom (*asraya*). Think of someone you consider a good friend and ask the following questions:

Sajatiya (like-minded)

How well does this person know your goals and aspirations in life, as well as the principles you try to live by? If this person was to give a eulogy of your life, how accurate and comprehensive would it be? Is this person easy to be around and have a conversation with?

Snehasya (affectionate)

In times of need, is your friend there for you? Does your friend make excuses, disappearing when it becomes convenient? Are you able to talk openly without fear of being misunderstood or judged? Can you disagree with this person and still feel close to them? Is this person genuinely happy in your success and looking for opportunities to help you achieve?

Asraya (shelter and help)

Has this person genuinely given you help which has improved and upgraded your life? Is this person someone you intuitively think of when you need help? Is this person able to give you critical feedback and openly talk about improvements that you need to make in your life?

Reflection

Pick one of your current friendships and, with reference to the three guiding principles above, state three things you could do today which would upgrade the relationship.

1.

2.

3.

13

I am
already happy!

Cruising through town in a high-end convertible, tinted windows and maxed-out subwoofers, lined with a windscreen caption which reads, *'Living the dream!'* People do feel like that: *"I have a snazzy car, two houses, great career, time for several holidays a year, beautiful family, and amazing health - what more could I ask for?"* Content with almost everything, they see spirituality as a fall-back for those who are missing abundance and achievement in their own lives.

In Chapter Thirteen, entitled 'Nature, the Enjoyer and Consciousness,' these subjects are analytically dissected. Krishna delineates two broad approaches to life. In the first, the soul (consciousness) selfishly exploits and enjoys nature, excommunicating God from the picture. In the second, the soul utilises the gifts of material nature in the service of God, seeing Him as the Supreme Enjoyer. According to the approach we adopt, we reap a certain quality of life. When we lack selfless spirituality and the sole objective becomes our own enjoyment of matter, despite the sprinkles of instant pleasure that periodically appear, we ultimately fall way short of the deep, fulfilling satisfaction that we seek so much.

In his paper, 'A Theory of Motivation,' Abraham Maslow established the now famous 'Hierarchy of Needs,' explaining how we're driven to pursue happiness on different levels. When basic needs are met, the human focuses on higher pursuits, seeking deeper and more subtle experiences. This continues through multiple stages, with the climax being 'self-actualisation' - the most satisfying state of human existence.

The model begins with the baseline necessities of human existence. We require food, clothing and shelter for survival, and until we're sufficiently equipped it's difficult to consider anything else. Once obtained, we strive for security and safety; a sense of cementing the future. With this in place, the individual next pursues emotional gratification through family, friendship, society, and meaningful exchange with others. Beyond that, one focuses on building their esteem and sense of self-worth through achievements, accolades and recognition in society. Having realised these four objectives, Maslow posited the ultimate endeavour to be 'self-actualisation.' Here, one's vision expands and they awaken their deeper purpose, inner-calling and authentic self. According to Maslow, only 2% of the world's population get anywhere near this stage.

Maslow's first four levels address the external coverings of the soul – the physical body, the mind, intelligence and ego. While we cannot ignore these very real needs, we must simultaneously understand that they're not the be all and end all of life. Thus, one of Krishna's striking recommendations in the Bhagavad-gita, which sounds counter-intuitive, is to *tolerate happiness*. We tolerate insult and criticism, reversals in the world, misfortunes of life – but why should we tolerate happiness? Isn't that feeling the very thing we're all looking for?

As we navigate life, varieties of physical and subtle pleasure can attract our attention and indulge our minds. These, Krishna says, should be 'tolerated,' since they only cater to the external coverings, the first four levels. If we become indulgent or content with such temporal delights we grab the shadow and miss the substance. Those who venture further, taste real happiness.

"The living entity in material nature thus follows the ways of life, enjoying the three modes of nature. This is due to his association with that material nature. Thus he meets with good and evil among various species."

(Bhagavad-gita 13.22)

References

13.21 – How the embodied soul attempts to enjoy in this material world.

13.24 – The development of pure spiritual consciousness.

Hierarchy of Needs

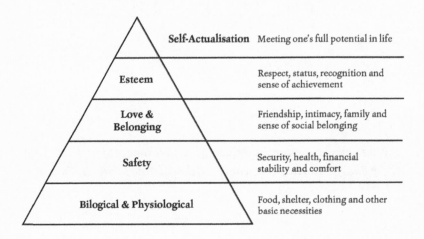

Based on the model above, ask yourself the following questions:

1) Which layer consumes most of your time, attention and energy? Why do you think that is and what could you do to change it?

2) *What has been your experience of happiness on the first four levels? Why do you think we continue to invest so much time in these aspects of life?*

3) *What does self-actualisation mean to you? From your understanding of the Bhagavad-gita, how would Krishna define self-actualisation?*

4) *What activities would help one become self-actualised?*

14

I have too many
bad habits

We sometimes look at ourselves and wish we were better, free of those behaviours and bad habits that plague us. *"I'm not a nice person,"* someone may say, *"and spirituality is for the noble and decent."* Responding to those who feel disqualified and unworthy, Krishna offers an encouraging perspective. Each and every soul in creation is pure, He says, but currently enveloped by material influences which inhibit that purity from shining through. Those influences come in the form of the three modes of nature, and practically everyone, to a greater or lesser extent, falls prey to that energy.

In Chapter Fourteen, Krishna discusses the three modes and delineates how they intricately intermix to trap the soul into an ever-mutating web of complex entanglement. Nobody is bad per se, just that we're covered by these superfluous influences. Spiritual practices empower us to 'rise above the clouds.' A crucial consideration, however, is that such practices are more effective and transformative when couched within spiritual lifestyle.

It's something like 'home advantage' in a football match. You're playing against the same players, running on the same grass, using the same ball, and trying to score in the same-sized goalposts. What's the difference? Well, history shows that having a familiar environment and encouraging crowd is nearly always a game-changer. Every football pundit will tell you – when you play at home, even before the whistle is blown, it's as if you're one goal up.

Spirituality is also easier when you have the home advantage. 'Home' consists of the right habits, diet, atmosphere and company. 'Home' means to live in *sattva*, the mode of goodness. To become completely selfless, humble, tolerant and naturally aligned with God is a lofty ideal. We can, however, gain momentum in that internal shift by diligently (and seemingly mechanically) making small but specific lifestyle adjustments. It's these finer details that we sometimes neglect, thinking them insignificant and unimportant in the bigger picture.

How clean is our environment? How regulated are we in habits of eating and sleeping? How mindful are we about the quality of our conversations? What are we willing to abstain from to preserve physical and emotional wellbeing? Pure action leads to pure mind which leads to pure consciousness. A spiritualist also needs to be a lifestyle engineer.

That lifestyle becomes the spiritual 'home ground' where it's easier to remember who you are and what your purpose really is. They say you can't change the beginning, but you can start where you are and change the end. Small, incremental and cumulative adjustments will create the bigger transformation of heart that we all seek. We may feel the process of change is slow, but rest assured, giving up won't make it any quicker!

It's a process of reengineering our 'inclination.' If you picture a tilted floor, whenever water drops down it naturally flows in a certain direction. In our current inclination, we have an easy time developing bad habits, but struggle to imbibe the good ones. Using the Gita's insights of the modes we can reengineer that inclination and begin effortlessly flowing towards the positive and beneficial, creating a life which unleashes our full potential.

"Sometimes the mode of goodness becomes prominent, defeating the modes of passion and ignorance, O son of Bharata. Sometimes the mode of passion defeats goodness and ignorance, and at other times ignorance defeats goodness and passion. In this way there is always competition for supremacy."

(Bhagavad-gita 14.10)

References

14.11-13 – Effects of the three modes.

14.26 – Rising above these three modes and becoming transcendental.

Four a Day

For an endeavouring spiritualist, four key areas of life are highlighted as being of paramount importance. Mark yourself out of ten on each of these areas and identify one thing you can do to improve that score.

1. Sleep

- Resting the body at a regulated time everyday

- Early to bed and early to rise

- 6-8 hours for sleep (adjust according to health / age)

- Sleeping on the right or left side, avoiding the stomach

Score (/10)

Improvements:

2. Diet

- Regular meal times, avoiding anything just before sleep

- Eat a balanced, fresh, vegetarian diet, offering that food in a spiritual way

- Opt for home-cooked food which is prepared with care and attention

- Incorporate fast days for giving the body a break / recuperation

Score (/10)

Improvements:

3. Cleanliness

- In one's environment – house, office, car

- In one's relationships – avoiding gossip, envy, criticism / being positive and empowering

- In physical habits – bodily, clothes, daily routines

- In consciousness – avoiding mental contemplations that compromise purity

Score (/10)

Improvements:

4. Meditation

- Establish as a daily practice

- Give your full focus and attention (no multi-tasking)

- Performed early morning, in a fresh, quiet environment

- Have a dedicated time in the year (perhaps a week or two) where you immerse yourself in a deeper way

Score (/10)

Improvements:

15

I'll lose my ambition and won't be successful

People often appreciate our spiritual interest at first, but when involvement grows, commitment deepens and priorities change, that's when the alarm bells start ringing! They welcome the morality and values that spirituality brings, but also develop a fear that we may become too detached from the world, lose our drive for success and renounce all ambitions for a prosperous future. *Can spirituality, philosophy and reflection make us so 'otherworldly' that we fail to harness the potential for success in the here and now?*

It's not that spiritualists lose the drive to succeed, but rather they redefine what constitutes success. Because the upgraded goals don't tally with people's stereotyped notions of achievement, it's assumed that spiritualists have retired from the race for success. In reality, they've re-invested their energy in something far more exciting, fulfilling and life-changing. Spiritualists let go of material ambitions not because they are faint-hearted, but because they are firmly determined. They turn away from those sought-after success symbols not because those things are too hard to obtain, but because they're too insignificant. Spiritualists widen their vision of success beyond their own achievements, selflessly empowering and serving everyone around them. They deepen their vision of success by seeking it on the most profound spiritual level.

In Chapter Fifteen, Krishna offers an entire paradigm shift of the world before us. Employing the metaphor of a reflected banyan tree, He explains how this world is simply a mirror image of the real form, the spiritual world which is situated in another dimension. *How can you find substance in a reflection, shadow, or photocopy of the original?* Spiritualists turn away from the ephemeral success of this world and turn their attention towards success of a different nature.

Srila Prabhupada was a mendicant, and also a wildly successful spiritual entrepreneur! When he arrived in America, he described the forty rupees he had with him as *"A few hours spending money in New York City."* Upon departing this world, ISKCON had grown to a worldwide organisation boasting hundreds of properties and unimaginable revenues. When he left India he had one disciple, by 1977 he had 5000. When he left India he had no temple established, after tirelessly traveling for 11 years he managed to open 108. When he left India it was his first time visiting foreign lands. Later, by the grace of Krishna, he circled the globe 14 times. Wherever there is Krishna and His sincere devotee, there will certainly be opulence and victory.

When CNN documented the top ten wildly successful people who activated their careers after the age of fifty, they included Srila Prabhupada in that elite list. What could be more ambitious than trying to trigger a revolution of consciousness so people can flourish on all levels - physically, emotionally, socially and spiritually. Srila Prabhupada's story is living proof that spiritualists can make the biggest impact, achieve the most astounding things and leave a lasting legacy for generations to come. They're not shooting stars, but rather effulgent moons which bring spiritual light to a dark world.

"This is the most confidential part of the Vedic scriptures, O sinless one, and it is disclosed now by Me. Whoever understands this will become wise, and his endeavours will know perfection."

(Bhagavad-gita 15.20)

References

15.7 - The struggle of the spirit soul in this world.

15.8 - The desires and activities of this life create one's next life.

Chasing Dreams

Can you think of an aspiration in your life which you managed to fulfil? Did it satisfy you, and what happened after you attained that success? How has your experience of 'success' in material achievements shaped your current goals?

List three aspirations you have at present. Upon reflection, if you do manage to fulfil them do you think they'll make you happy? If not, why are they still so important for you to achieve?

I see how religion causes more problems

Recent world events have compounded apprehensions about the social implications of religious belief. While governments grapple with the problem of terrorism, the growing opposition to religion becomes strikingly apparent. As a travelling monk, I'm often drawn into heated debates over the link between religion and war. To complicate matters further, the Bhagavad-gita is spoken at the onset of fratricidal battle, and Krishna is the one encouraging Arjuna to fight! *Does the Bhagavad-gita promote bloodshed and violence? Do spiritualists in this tradition secretly believe that aggression, hostility and the killing of innocent people are necessary for 'religious revolution'? Wouldn't the world be a more peaceful place without religion?*

As a guardian of society, Arjuna was duty-bound to safeguard law and order. In this case, his non-violence had to be expressed through confrontational means. To passively withdraw would be to neglect those who required his care and protection. Such strong action is neither taken whimsically, nor for the sake of selfish gain, and never with a mood of bitterness, hatred or envy. It was the last resort, and even when the battle commenced, it was fought between consenting parties who honoured strict moral and ethical codes of warfare. Before drawing any parallels between the Battle of Kuruksetra and modern-day conflicts, we have to understand the historical, cultural and social context of each situation.

Violence has touched every part of the world, religious or otherwise. In fact, the most destructive wars were driven by secular, political or economic reasons. Admittedly, however, religion can become dogmatic and decadent, manipulated to fuel war, violence and friction in the world. True religion should give birth to genuine spiritualists who hold sacred reverence for life - respect, contentment, humility and tolerance are the cardinal principles they live by.

In Chapter Sixteen, Krishna discusses divine and demoniac tendencies, and identifies the root cause of unrest in society. When people embrace the idea that the world is unreal, with no God in control (*asatyam anisvaram*), and that it appears from a random interaction of nature (*kama-haitukam*), they pave the path toward destruction. By removing God from the picture they become lost to themselves, unaware of their spiritual identity (*nastatmano*). In such ignorance they can't truly perceive the equality of all living beings, and thus engage in unbeneficial, destructive work (*ugra karma*) meant to ruin the world (*ksayaya jagat*). It's not a pretty picture.

Far from fuelling the problem, pure spirituality is the only real solution. Ignorance plus money equals corruption. Ignorance plus power equals dictatorship. Ignorance plus freedom equals anarchy. Ignorance plus religion equals terrorism. You'll notice the common element in every equation - ignorance. The problem is not the thing, but the ignorance which causes people to misuse that thing. Despite the disturbances caused by inauthentic, misguided religionists, we should be careful not to dismiss religion in its entirety. The greatest need in today's world is genuine spiritualists who embody genuine purity. This is the only hope for bringing people together in an otherwise disunited and disharmonious world.

"They say that this world is unreal, with no foundation, no God in control. They say it is produced of sex desire and has no cause other than lust. Following such conclusions, the demoniac, who are lost to themselves and who have no intelligence, engage in unbeneficial, horrible works meant to destroy the world."

(Bhagavad-gita 16.8-9)

References

16.9 – The destructive effects of atheistic philosophy.

Spiritual Solutions

Look at the five major categories of problems below. Can you explain how each one may have its roots in a lack of spirituality? How would the promotion of spiritual values in society help to solve these problems?

Environmental Problems – scarce natural resources, pollution, unbalanced ecosystem, extinct species

Economic Problems – rich-poor gap, debt, distribution of wealth in world, unstable economies

Social Problems - crime, prostitution, antisocial behaviour, racism, sexism, nationalism

Individual Problems - mental illness, physical illness, teenage pregnancy, addictions

Global Problems - war, terrorism, natural disasters

17

I've seen too much
hypocrisy in religion

Meeting people on high streets, showing them wisdom books and trying to spark some spiritual interest is something I did for many years. You have a twenty-second window to make an impression – they stop, you gather your wits, put in a spiritual pitch, something interesting, inspirational and endearing, and wait for a reaction – hit, miss or blank... anything could happen! Interestingly, people are more perceptive than we may think. They can sniff out any sense of superficiality, personal agenda, self-righteousness or insecurity within moments. Often they'll make it known to you, and boy is that humbling! Other times they stay quiet, but it leaves an impression on them. People may forget what you say, but they'll never forget how you made them feel. One striking life lesson I've learnt is that teachers can't be cheaters.

For many, spiritual teachings make complete sense, but a block remains. When they see a major gap between the revered teachings and the conduct of the practitioners, it raises serious doubts. Everyone wants to see spiritualists who walk the talk and practice what they preach.

In Chapter Seventeen, entitled 'Divisions of Faith,' Krishna reveals that any given activity can be performed by multiple individuals, each harbouring a different mindset and motivation. Thus, we can't be utopian in our vision even amongst those who practice spirituality. There are gradations of purity within any given group.

Don't we witness lies, hypocrisy and cheating in all aspects of life? A shop may advertise a half-price sale. After purchasing a product you may think you've *saved* £500 but the reality is that they've ingeniously induced you into *spending* £500! Shops are cheating, yet we continue buying products. Politicians are regularly compromised, yet we still vote for one of them. The media spreads misinformation, but we still read newspapers.

It's unrealistic to expect 100% purity in anything of this world, and we should bear this in mind when seeking a spiritual path to tread. Instead of focusing on the deficient practitioners, we'd do well to seek out the serious and sincere ones who live with integrity. Look closely enough and you'll find many who are living examples of purity.

It was Gandhi who famously reminded us to *"Be the change we want to see in the world."* The challenge is for us to become examples of purity, and that journey begins with honesty. Instead, however, we are often closed and pretentious. In the name of saving our face, we kill our soul. Sometimes we invent, sometimes we withhold, sometimes we exaggerate and sometimes we stay quiet and let the lies roll - a variety of ingenious ways in which we compromise our integrity. It's scary to think how much of our day can be spent lying - rehearsing future conversations, reconfiguring events of the past and reinforcing inaccurate perceptions of the present. We all know the value of meditation, yoga and study in our spiritual growth. Let us, however, not underestimate some of the more fundamental disciplines and human qualities that can prove equally valuable in this profound journey. Truthfulness is definitely one of them.

"O son of Bharata, according to one's existence under the various modes of nature, one evolves a particular kind of faith. The living being is said to be of a particular faith according to the modes he has acquired."

(Bhagavad-gita 17.3)

References

17.4 - varieties of worship in different modes.

17.14-17 - austerities of those following true spirituality.

The Truth about Lying

The hypocrisy and duplicity of others screams out to us, but if we're honest, such imperfections also exist within us. The great saint Bhaktisiddhanta Saraswati Thakur once said: *"When faults in others misguide and delude you, have patience, introspect - find faults in yourself. Know that others cannot harm you unless you harm yourself."*

Reflect on the last week and try to identify a situation in which you:

Said something untrue:

Purposely witheld information to misguide others:

Exaggerated a truth so it ended up a lie:

Avoided speaking the truth when you could have:

Can you think of the three main reasons why you lie and how can you overcome those factors?

18

I don't want to be
forced

We've reached the conclusion. A multitude of excuses have been presented, and a series of responses offered. There could still, however, be one final reservation. Though everything may make sound logical sense, we still have to embrace it from within. *"I can't force it"* someone may say *"I have to do it from the heart."*

Krishna fully agrees. After speaking many verses, presenting a flawless philosophy, and patiently addressing all of Arjuna's questions, confusions and doubts, Krishna humbly states that this wisdom is merely *"His opinion"* and that Arjuna should *"reflect upon the conversation, weigh up the options, and then do as he wishes to do."* The Bhagavad-gita thus concludes with a resounding emphasis on free will - a gift of God that He never impinges upon. *Bhakti* is an affair of the heart.

Every year I travel to the beautiful village of Vrindavana, the home of Krishna, for a boost of spiritual inspiration and rejuvenation. A casual stroll through the dusty lanes reveals a depth of wisdom. Holy places are invaluable because they're a living theology; what's written about in pages of books and discussed in hours of discourses, is lucidly revealed in the simple and sincere lifestyle of devotion that comes so naturally to the people there.

I make a point to visit the Radha Damodara Temple, where Srila Prabhupada spent many reflective years before coming to America. During his time there, he observed a Bengali widow who devotedly walked to the Yamuna River every morning, returning with a clay pot of sacred water for the daily temple worship. Sometimes he would open the gate for her, intently noting her demeanour. Moved by her devotion, he said she would surely attain spiritual perfection in this very life, her entrance to eternity guaranteed, for her heart was completely devoid of selfishness and pretention. She had grasped the essence – that she was a spirit soul, and the most valuable opportunity in life was to connect with the Supreme Spirit through love and service in whatever simple way she could. A natural devotion from deep within.

Even today, we encounter many saintly souls in Vrindavana. They live as lone mendicants in the holy land, probably with a vow to never leave, determined to end their days in complete spiritual absorption, diligently preparing for their imminent journey to the next world. They have understood this is the business end of life – where the greatest opportunities open up.

It always prompts me to reflect on the intensity of my own spirituality. We have to build momentum, increase the urgency and eagerly look for more and more avenues to genuinely go deeper. Gradually, all the empty promises of the world that steal our attention should fade into insignificance, allowing us to focus on the essence of life.

After much discussion, the ball, as they say, really is in our court. While one remains on the philosophical platform, there will always be a ping-pong of arguments to consider. Doubts will linger and hesitancy will remain. To become truly convinced one must progress beyond the intellectual. The higher dimensional methodology involves a transcendental exchange with Krishna. That is the greatest challenge and the greatest opportunity that the Bhagavad-gita offers to us all. We have to make the step, and we have to make it with our heart.

"Thus I have explained to you knowledge still more confidential. Deliberate on this fully, and then do what you wish to do."

(Bhagavad-gita 18.63)

References

18.63 – Krishna encourages Arjuna to exercise his free will.

18.66 – Krishna's final piece of advice to Arjuna, encouraging a heartfelt surrender.

12 months, 12 goals!

In this book we've discussed various philosophical points, conducted numerous thought experiments, reflected on our lives, character and inner world, and gathered tips and techniques of spiritual empowerment. Now knowledge has to be transformed into action.

On the worksheet opposite you can write 12 goals for the 12 coming months and practically visualise how you'll progressively achieve those goals.

Try to ensure that each goal is SMART:

S - Specific

M - Measurable

A - Attainable

R - Relevant

T - Time based

	Months 1-4	Months 5-8	Months 9-12
Spirituality My goals in studying wisdom and practicing meditation	*e.g. Finish Reading the entire Bhagavad-gita in 4 months*		
Character My goals in transforming and developing my character			
Contribution My goals to selflessly serve others and contribute to a better world			
Other My miscellaneous goals (e.g. exercise, relationships)			

Summary | Why Not

If the very purpose of this world is to help the soul reawaken its original consciousness, it's logical to assume that not only can there be no impediments to spiritual progress, but rather everything in life can be favourably engaged towards that end. Justifications to deny or delay our spiritual progress are ultimately nothing more than excuses. We have the choice to expose and overcome them now, else it'll become apparent in hindsight, by which time those excuses will have given birth to many regrets. Overcoming excuses is uncomfortable, but living with regret is unbearable.

Appendix

Bhakti: The Yoga of Love

The heart yearns to experience love. Interestingly, when I became a monk I never imagined talking about love as much as I do! The stereotypical depiction of monasticism is solitude, renunciation, inner life, and a sense of withdrawal from everyone and everything. While many of those elements are definitely factored in, they don't constitute the goal. Without doubt, everyone looks for love – even monks! The problem, however, is that we generally equate love with romantic love. The Bhagavad-gita, however, introduces us to a transcendent perspective of love which is so all-encompassing that it spreads everywhere, in all directions, and pervades every aspect of our being. This love is divine love, awakened through the process of *bhakti-yoga*.

"Out of many thousands among men, one may endeavour for perfection, and of those who have achieved perfection, hardly one knows Me in truth." (Bhagavad-gita 7.3)

In Gita3 we have presented some of the most powerful philosophy, insightful psychology and everyday practicality that the Bhagavad-gita has to offer. Yet its ultimate contribution goes beyond the body, mind and intellect. The Gita's essential aim is to delineate various processes of *yoga*, or methods of spiritual connection. Krishna offers a variety of options, an ingenious yoga-ladder which gives everyone an entrance point to step up and elevate themselves. That progression culminates in *bhakti-yoga*, which combines and synthesises all other *yoga* processes. *Bhakti-yoga* awakens the soul's pure relationship of love with Krishna, the all-attractive Supreme Person.

"And of all yogis, the one with great faith who always abides in Me, thinks of Me within himself, and renders transcendental loving service to Me—he is the most intimately united with Me in yoga and is the highest of all. That is My opinion." (Bhagavad-gita 6.47)

The practice of *bhakti-yoga* and the journey of spiritual progression has been documented by the great spiritual preceptors of the

Gaudiya Vaisnava sampradaya, an ancient tradition of knowledge which remains fully intact even today. In the Bhakti-Rasmrita Sindhu, a 16th Century thesis on the science of devotion, the great teacher Rupa Goswami perfectly outlines the means to incorporate *bhakti-yoga* into one's daily life. Those teachings were brought into the modern light through the life and teachings of A.C. Bhaktivedanta Swami Prabhupada, the foremost exponent of the *bhakti* tradition throughout the entire world. Srila Prabhupada's own students contributed to the discourse by further expanding on the application of *bhakti* in contemporary, postmodern society, and their insights are also valuable.

Bhakti-yoga is practiced in many ways – through music, dance, selfless service, wisdom, worship and art, to name just a few. Since *bhakti-yoga* allows one to utilise their natural propensities for the purpose of spiritual elevation, it is considered the most practical and accessible path available. The path of devotion is best practiced with discipline and dedication (*vaidhi*), which eventually leads to a natural spontaneity (*raganuga*) in which there is effortless and uninterrupted experience of love. The study of *bhakti-yoga* is vast, but here we outline four fundamental aspects which form the basis of one's *bhakti Life*:

Association

We all need friends. On the journey of life there are twists and turns, ditches and dead ends, obstacles and opposition. But as John Lennon sang "*I get by with a little help from my friends.*" Those who embark on the spiritual journey are brave indeed. They strive for purity in a world of degradation, they embrace simplicity amongst rampant materialism, and they cultivate selflessness in an atmosphere charged with exploitation. Anyone who boldly goes against the grain will face temptation, doubt, ridicule and moments of weakness. The encouragement, support and good advice of spiritual friends is absolutely essential. Srila Prabhupada established ISKCON (International Society for Krishna Consciousness) to give people the chance to develop relationships with devotees of Krishna. This is one of the most effective ways to gain faith and become enthusiastic in spiritual life.

Tip: Try to visit a local ISKCON temple on a regular basis and take advantage of the classes, events and various opportunities for devotional service. If you live far away from a temple, you can attend one of the Krishna groups that meet regularly in various localities. At these gatherings, you can enjoy uplifting chanting, a lively and informative talk and prasadam (sanctified vegetarian food).

Books

There is nothing in this world as sublime as transcendental knowledge. Knowledge is compared to a sword which cuts down our doubts and helps one remain determined and confident in the spiritual quest. Knowledge is also likened to a lamp which warns us of the obstacles and impediments that we may encounter on that journey. In another metaphor, Krishna depicts knowledge as a boat which protects one from the sufferings of this oceanic world, simultaneously carrying one to the spiritual realm, face-to-face with Krishna. When Srila Prabhupada spoke into a Dictaphone and translated the timeless wisdom of the Vedas, Lord Krishna and the great teachers spoke through him. That spiritual sound was then transformed into the printed word, which, when read and assimilated, can once again manifest the full potency of the original sound.

Tip: Read the books translated by Srila Prabhupada. Along with the well-known Bhagavad-gita there is also the Srimad Bhagavatam. Its 18,000 verses continue the philosophical teachings of the Gita and also describe Krishna's divine appearance and incarnations. Srila Prabhupada also published the Caitanya Caritamrita, the biography and detailed teachings of Sri Chaitanya Mahaprabhu, Krishna's most recent incarnation. There are also the important works of Srila Rupa Goswami, medieval disciple of Sri Chaitanya, such as Bhakti Rasamrita Sindhu and Upadeshamrita.

Chanting

Five hundred years ago, Krishna incarnated as Sri Chaitanya Mahaprabhu and ushered in a spiritual revolution by freely inviting everyone – regardless of race, religion, or social status – into the chanting of the most effective *mantra* of all, the Hare Krishna *mantra*. Since God is all-powerful and all-merciful, He has kindly made it very easy for us to chant His names, and He has also invested all His powers in them. This means that when we chant the holy names of Krishna we are directly associating with Him and simultaneously being purified by such communion. Chanting is a prayer to Krishna that means *'O energy of the Lord (Hare), O all-attractive Lord (Krishna), O supreme enjoyer (Rama), please engage me in Your service.'* This chanting is exactly like the genuine cry of a child for its mother's presence.

Tip: Recite the Hare Krishna mantra on a circle of 108 wooden beads. This is known as japa meditation. One time round the beads each day is for beginners, four times round as a daily minimum is for more committed practitioners, and sixteen 'rounds' are for those who have taken (or are planning to take) their lifetime vows. You can chant these holy names of the Lord anywhere and at any time, but the early morning hours are deemed ideal.

Diet

The Bhagavad-gita declares eating to be an extremely sacred activity when conducted with due care, attention and spiritual consciousness. If we place an iron rod in fire, the rod quickly becomes red hot and acts just like fire. Similarly, food prepared for and offered to Krishna with love and devotion becomes completely spiritualised. Such food is called Krishna *prasadam*, which means *"the mercy of Lord Krishna."* Eating *prasadam* is a fundamental practice of *bhakti-yoga*. In other forms of *yoga* one must artificially repress the senses, but the *bhakti-yogi* can engage his or her senses in a variety of pleasing spiritual activities.

Tip: It is recommended that one offer their food to Krishna before eating. From the purchase of the ingredients, to the cooking, then the offering and finally the eating, every step can be an act of love which brings one closer to God. The process starts with selecting ingredients, those which are vegetarian, natural and fresh. In preparing food, cleanliness, attention and devotion are the main principles. After cooking, arrange portions of the food on special dinner-ware kept especially for Krishna. The easiest way to offer food is simply to pray, "My dear Lord Krishna, please accept this humble offering". There are also special mantras which can be chanted to invoke a devotional consciousness. Then you can accept that sanctified food and share it with others!

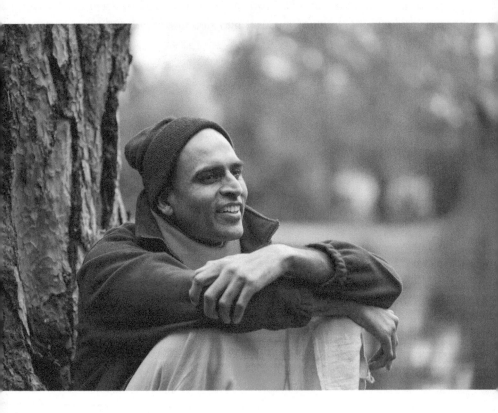

Author

Svayam Bhagavan Keshava Swami (S.B. Keshava Swami) is a spiritual author, community mentor, dynamic teacher and worldwide traveller. In 2002, after graduating from UCL (University College London) with a BSc in Information Management, he adopted full-time monastic life to expand his knowledge, deepen his spirituality and share these timeless principles with the wider society.

For over twenty years, Keshava Swami was a resident monk at ISKCON UK's headquarters, Bhaktivedanta Manor. There he pioneered the School of Bhakti, led the monastic training programme and drove forward national outreach projects. He has designed numerous courses on Vedic theology, lifestyle management and spiritual self-development, and has also authored numerous books which bring the ancient wisdom into the modern context.

In 2022, Keshava Swami accepted vows of lifetime renunciation. Nowadays he is a globe-trotter, teaching in universities, corporate firms, government organisations and spiritual communities, bringing wisdom to the places which need it the most. He continues to diligently study the Sanskrit texts, considering how to proliferate spiritual wisdom in a world that is suffocating from materialism.

Books by S.B. Keshava Swami

- Gita Life: A Summary of Bhagavad-gita

- IQ, EQ, SQ: Life, the Universe and Everything

- Tattva: See Inside Out

- Tattva2: Old Words Open New Worlds

- Bhakti Life: 18 Simple Steps to Krishna

- Chaitanya-Charitamrita Compact

- Book Bhagavata: The Life Companion

- Gita3: A Contemporary Guide to the Timeless Teachings of the Bhagavad-gita

- Playground of God

- Loving Life, Embracing Death

- Masterminds of Bhakti (Upcoming)

Books Compiled by S.B. Keshava Swami:

- Veda: Secrets of the East (A.C. Bhaktivedanta Swami Prabhupada)

- In Essence (A.C. Bhaktivedanta Swami Prabhupada)

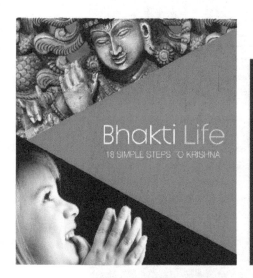

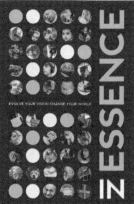

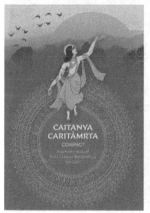

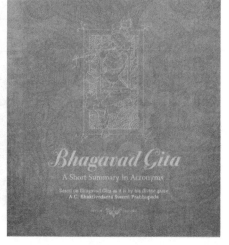

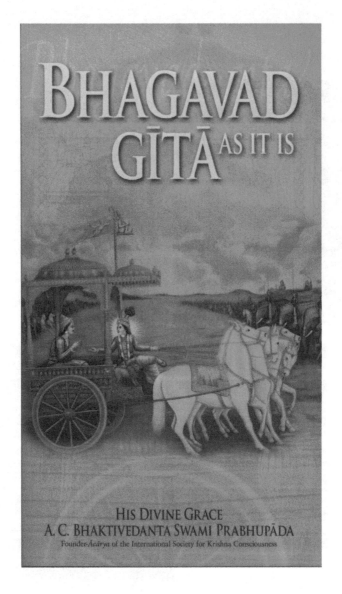

BHAGAVAD GĪTĀ AS IT IS

HIS DIVINE GRACE
A. C. BHAKTIVEDANTA SWAMI PRABHUPĀDA
Founder-Ācārya of the International Society for Krishna Consciousness

Read Bhagavad-gita As It Is online

www.vedabase.io

Made in the USA
Las Vegas, NV
15 September 2023

77600427R00131